Warts
Diagnosis and Management: An Evidence-based Approach

Warts
Diagnosis and Management
An Evidence-based Approach

Edited by

Robert T Brodell MD
Professor of Internal Medicine,
Clinical Professor of Dermatopathology in Pathology,
Master Teacher, Northeastern Ohio Universities College of Medicine
Rootstown, Ohio
Associate Clinical Professor of Dermatology,
Case Western Reserve University School of Medicine
Cleveland, Ohio
USA

Sandra Marchese Johnson MD
Director Dermatology Clinical Trials and
Assistant Professor, Department of Dermatology
University of Arkansas for Medical Sciences
Central Arkansas Veterans Healthcare System and
Arkansas Children's Hospital
Little Rock, Arkansas
USA

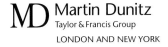 Martin Dunitz
Taylor & Francis Group
LONDON AND NEW YORK

© 2003 Martin Dunitz, a member of the Taylor & Francis Group

First published in the United Kingdom in 2003
by Martin Dunitz, Taylor & Francis Group plc, 11 New Fetter Lane, London EC4P 4EE

Tel: +44 (0) 20 7583 9855
Fax: +44 (-) 20 7842 2298
E-mail: info@dunitz.co.uk
Website: http://www.dunitz.co.uk

Although every effort has been made to ensure that all owners of copyright material have been acknowledged in this publication, we would be glad to acknowledge in subsequent reprints or editions any omissions brought to our attention.

Although every effort has been made to ensure that drug doses and other information are presented accurately in this publication, the ultimate responsibility rests with the prescribing physician. Neither the publishers nor the authors can be held responsible for errors or for any consequences arising from the use of information contained herein. For detailed prescribing information or instructions on the use of any product or procedure discussed herein, please consult the prescribing information or instructional material issued by the manufacturer.

A CIP record for this book is available from the British Library.

ISBN 1 84184 240 0

Distributed in the USA by
Fulfilment Center
Taylor & Francis
10650 Tobben Drive
Independence, KY 41051, USA
Toll free tel: +1 800 634 7064
E-mail: taylorandfrancis@thomsonlearning.com

Distributed in Canada by
Taylor & Francis
74 Rolark Drive
Scarborough, Ontario M1R 4G2, Canada
Toll free tel: +1 877 226 2237
E-mail: tal_fran@istar.ca

Distributed in the rest of the world by
Thomson Publishing Services
Cheriton House
North Way
Andover, Hampshire SP10 5BE, UK
Tel: +44 (0) 1264 332424
E-mail: salesorder.tandf@thomsonpublishingservices.co.uk

Composition by Scribe Design, Gillingham, Kent, UK
Printed and bound in Spain by Grafos S.A. Arte Sobre Papel

Contents

CONTENTS

List of contributors

Pradip Bhattacharjee
Pathology
Forum Health
Youngstown, Ohio
and Pathology
Northeastern Ohio Universities College of
Medicine
Rootstown, Ohio
USA

Robert T Brodell
Professor of Internal Medicine, Clinical
Professor of Dermatopathology in Pathology,
Master Teacher, Northeastern Ohio
Universities College of Medicine
Rootstown, Ohio
Associate Clinical Professor of Dermatology,
Case Western Reserve University School of
Medicine
Cleveland, Ohio
USA

Jessica Causbie Pillow
Department of Dermatology
University of Arkansas for Medical Sciences
Little Rock, Arkansas
USA

Susannah Lambird Collier
Department of Dermatology
University of Arkansas for Medical Sciences
Central Arkansas Veterans Healthcare System
and Arkansas Children's Hospital
Little Rock, Arkansas
USA

Charles Davis
Department of Dermatology
University of Arkansas for Medical Sciences
Little Rock, Arkansas
USA

Geneviève Fortier-Riberdy
Department of Dermatology
University of Arkansas for Medical Sciences
Little Rock, Arkansas
USA

Fareedah Goodwin
Northeastern Ohio Universities College of
Medicine
Rootstown, Ohio
USA

Amy Helms
Washington and Jefferson College
Washington, Pennsylvania
USA

Stephen E Helms
Associate Professor of Clinical Internal
Medicine, Northeastern Ohio Universities
College of Medicine
Rootstown, Ohio
Assistant Clinical Professor of Dermatology,
Case Western Reserve University School of
Medicine
Cleveland, Ohio
USA

Walter Hubert
Assistant Professor
Department of Dermatology
University of Arkansas for Medical Sciences
Little Rock, Arkansas
USA

Sandra Marchese Johnson
Director Dermatology Clinical Trials and
Assistant Professor
Department of Dermatology
University of Arkansas for Medical Sciences
Central Arkansas Veterans Healthcare System
and Arkansas Children's Hospital
Little Rock, Arkansas
USA

Manish Khanna
Department of Dermatology
University of Arkansas for Medical Sciences
Little Rock, Arkansas
USA

Angeline F Lim
Northeastern Ohio Universities College of
Medicine
Rootstown, Ohio
USA

Huwaida E Mansour
Department of Internal Medicine
Forum Health
Northside Medical Center
Youngstown, Ohio
USA

E Brian Russell
Department of Dermatology
University of Arkansas for Medical Sciences
Central Arkansas Veterans Healthcare System
and Arkansas Children's Hospital
Little Rock, Arkansas
USA

Geeta Mohla Shah
Case Western Reserve University School of
Medicine
Cleveland, Ohio
USA

Sanjay Sheth
American University of the Caribbean
St Maarten, Netherland Antilles

Zulma I Toledo
Forum Health
Tod Children's Hospital
Youngstown, Ohio and
Ponce School of Medicine
Ponce, Puerto Rico

Kyle L Wagamon IV
Case Western Reserve University School of
Medicine
Cleveland, Ohio
USA

Brian S Wayne
Department of Dermatology,
University of Arkansas for Medical Sciences
Little Rock, Arkansas
USA

Maria Lindsey Wirges
Department of Dermatology,
University of Arkansas for Medical Sciences
Little Rock, Arkansas
USA

Preface

Dermatologists are confronted with many vexing problems in their clinical work, but the patient with the 'thousand dollar' wart is one of the most frustrating. These warts resist multiple treatments and stress bot the patient and physician. Tailoring treatment to each individual patient, involving the patient in decisions regarding their care, understanding the wide range of available modalities, and basing treatment on available scientific evidence, leads to positive results in the vast majority of even the most difficult cases.

In producing this book we stand on the shoulders of our mentors who taught us the science of medicine. These individuals include William L. Morgan, M.D., George Engle, M.D., Arthur Z. Eisen, M.D., Eugene A. Bauer, M.D., Blake J. Goslen, M.D., Daniel J. Santa Cruz, M.D., David R. Bickers, M.D., Thomas D. Horn, M.D. and Robert T. Brodell, M.D. (for Sandra Marchese Johnson). The second key ingredient was the unwavering support of our loving families. We would like to acknowledge our parents, siblings, spouses and children, and the staff at our workplaces who have become our extended family. This book is also dedicated to our students, past, present, and future.

Robert T. Brodell, Ohio
Sandra Marchese Johnson, Arkansas

Part I
Background

1 Warts and all

Brian S Wayne and Sandra Marchese Johnson

Of all the futile disorders of the skin, it would be hard to find any that are regarded with greater contempt by the lay public and yet capable of resisting a greater variety of treatment than the group of papillary lesions commonly known as warts.[1]

This statement made by Lempière in 1951 shows the great impact that warts have had on society over the millennia. Warts have afflicted humankind at least since the times of ancient Greece and Rome, and currently can be found in literature, art, movies and other areas of society.

The Greeks and Romans were the first to use terms describing warts. The word condyloma is of Greek origin and means knuckle or knob. Myrmecia is a term derived from the Greek word for anthill. The term verruca was first used by Sennertus and originally meant a steep place or height. In Roman–Hellenistic times, genital warts were referred to using the terms 'ficus' and 'thymus'. Ficus, a Latin word meaning fig, was originally used as an obscene word. This word was chosen because the Romans believed that a group of warts resembled the inside of a cut-open fig. The word thymus is also a Latin word, derived from the Greek word *thymos* or *thymion*, which was used because of the similarities in the appearance of genital warts to the tips of the thyme plant.[2,3] Romans were aware that genital warts could be sexually transmitted.[4] Early Hippocratic writings also refer to 'pedunculated warts' occurring in children. Celsus, in AD 25 in his work on medicine *De Medicina*, mentions three types of wart-like lesions:

One kind the Greeks call acrochordon, wherein is the development of something hard and uneven under the skin, the latter retaining its natural colour. It is thin towards its extremity, but broad at its base, and of moderate size, rarely exceeding a bean in dimensions. It is seldom solitary, but commonly occurs in clusters, and principally in children. Sometimes these little tumours terminate on a sudden; but at other times they become inflamed and are removed by suppuration. Another kind they call thymion – a little wart which projects considerably from the skin, slender at the base, broad, hard and uneven, and coloured at its summit like the blossom of the thyme, from which peculiarity it derives its name. The thymion splits up easily at the summit and is raw, and sometimes it bleeds a little; its ordinary size is that of an Egyptian bean, rarely bigger, sometimes extremely small. Sometimes it occurs singly; sometimes there are several, and both in the palms

*and in the soles of the feet. The worst
kind are those which are developed about
the organs of generation; and there they
bleed more freely than elsewhere.
Myrmecia is the name given to warts
dwarfer and harder then the thymion. Their
roots are deeper; they are more painful;
they are broader at the base then at the
summit; they are less disposed to bleed;
and they hardly ever exceed the
dimensions of a lupin in size. They are
met with in the palms of the hands and
the soles of the feet.'*

The descriptions show that Celsus recognized molluscum contagiosum, genital warts and common warts, respectively.[2–4]

There have been multiple ideas on the aetiology of warts throughout the ages. Original lay ideas of aetiology included repeated wetting of the hands, washing the hands in water in which eggs had been boiled, the foam of the sea-shore, the killing of a toad (where the person would develop as many warts as the toad had spots), masturbation, and contact with cows or chickens.[2,5,6] Some people believed that the appearance of a wart on the right hand was a sign that foretold sickness.[5,6] In 1712, Daniel Turner suggested that warts might be 'congealed nutritious juices' that had seeped from damaged nerve filaments in the skin.[3,7] Dr Durr in an article from *The Lancet* in 1849 'maintained that females addicted to solitary habits (masturbation) often present with warts of the index and middle fingers'.[2,6] Our current superstition about the cause of warts is that the urine of a frog or toad will cause warts if it touches the skin.

The start of discovering the truth about the aetiology began in 1823 when Sir Astley Cooper stated, 'I must observe, that they frequently secrete a matter which is able to produce a similar disease in others'.[2] Joseph Payne, in 1891, recorded the contagious nature of warts when he described how he developed a wart under his thumbnail one week after treating an 11-year-old boy. Payne softened the warts with salicylic and acetic acids and then scraped them away, once using his thumbnail. He stated, 'Common warts ... appear to arise by the implantation of some contagious material at one or more points of the skin, usually on exposed parts'.[2,3,5,7] In 1894 Variot inoculated warts from a child to an adult and Jadassohn confirmed the infective nature of warts by his own inoculation experiments. The probable viral origin of warts was suggested by the work of Ciuffo in 1907. He produced warts on his hands by inoculating himself with a wart extract that had passed through a Berkefeld filter with a pore size that excluded bacteria and fungi. In 1949 Strauss et al were the first to visualize viral particles in warts by using electron microscopy. Melnick then classified the wart virus into the Papova virus group in 1962.[2,3,5–7]

Folk cures for warts were many. One of the earliest recorded treatments is from Celsus who suggested burning warts away with the ash of wine-lees.[7] During the first century Galen mentions a 'dextrous fellow' who went about biting or sucking off verruca and myrmecia from the feet of sufferers. In the sixteenth century Sir Francis Bacon claims to have cured his warts by rubbing them with pork fat that was then hung in the sun – as the fat melted the warts disappeared.[3,7] He also mentions curing warts by rubbing them with a green alder stick, which was then buried and allowed to rot, taking the warts with it. In the seventeenth century Sir Kenelm Digby reported a cure for warts by 'washing the hands in moonbeams, in an otherwise empty, well-polished, silver basin'.[5,6] Daniel Turner, in 1712 in his medical text *De Morbis Cutaneis*, discusses application of plant extracts, paring with a sharp penknife and the use of corrosives such as brimstone as wart cures.[7]

DA Burns' article in the *Journal of the Royal Society of Medicine* (1992) suggests that folk cures could be categorized as follows: (1) transference; (2) animal, plant or mineral remedies; (3) prayers and incantations (usually in association with above); (4) miscellaneous cures; and (5) any combination of the above.[2] Although Burns was the most recent to categorize these cures, William George Black, in his book on folk medicine published in 1883, also suggests nine categories similar to those of Burns, with transference again at the top of the list.[8] Transference seemed to be the most popular method for curing warts. Warts could be transferred to another person, a plant or an inanimate object, either directly or through an intermediary object.[2,5] One example is to rub the warts against a man who is the father of an illegitimate child. When this is done without his knowledge, the warts are speedily removed.[2,5,6,8] There are also reports of vagrants who would agree to take away a person's warts by having them count the number of warts and write this on the inside of his hat.[2,5,6,9] This was done for a small consideration of course. Rubbing the warts with the hand of a corpse could also cure warts.[8] Another way to complete a transference was to rub the warts with a cinder that was then tied up in paper and dropped at a crossroads. When another person picked up and opened the packet, this would transfer the warts to that person. This theme also applies to putting pebbles, equal in number to warts, into a bag and throwing the bag over the left shoulder to wait for an unexpecting person to pick the bag up. There is also evidence of transference via sale, if you could find someone charitable enough to purchase them; the price does not seem to matter.[2,5,6,8]

Transference can also occur to other living creatures. One cure occurs by rubbing a living black-shelled snail on each wart for a period of nine consecutive days and then hanging the snail on a thorn, with or without speaking the incantation, 'Wart wart, on the snail's shell black, Go away soon, and never come back'. When the snail rots the warts disappear.[2,6,8–10] Another way to cure warts was to impale a toad on a stick and rub the warts on the creature. As the toad dies the warts will disappear.[9] Cats can also be used, living or dead. The advice of Huckleberry Finn in *The Adventures of Tom Sawyer* is, 'Say – what is dead cats good for Huck? Good for. Cure warts with'.[11] Transference to the ash tree was also popular. This was accomplished by rubbing the warts with a piece of bacon and then placing the bacon into a slit cut into the bark of the tree. The warts would soon disappear from your hand and reappear on the tree as areas of excrescences or knobs. An alternative cure is to stick a pin into the ash tree, into the wart, and then into the tree again, leaving it there. This ritual was performed while repeating the words 'Ashen tree, Ashen tree, Pray buy these warts of me'.[2,5,6,8] In addition, elderberry leaves plucked at midnight and burnt were suggested to drive warts away.[9] An example of transference to an inanimate object was to 'Take a piece of worsted and tie in it as many knots as you have warts, and then drop this down the lavatory'. As the worsted decayed the warts were supposed to disappear.[2,5,6]

Remedies were numerous and have included fish heads, pig's blood, pig's fat, lizard's blood, menstrual blood, dog's dung, dove's dung, tobacco juice and fasting saliva.[2,6,8] Bleiberg mentions a grade school teacher in Newark, New Jersey, who cured the warts of her pupils by having them apply their own saliva. This had to be done in the morning before they brushed their teeth because toothpaste was said to kill the wart-destroying factor.[2,12] Other suggestions have been scorpion heads, mole's blood and a piece of one's own skin.[5,6] *Culpeper's Complete Herbal* (1652) includes buckthorn, houseleek and celandine as plant remedies for warts.[2] Ross mentions taking the entrails of a freshly killed hen and wrapping them around the area of the warts. Once this is done the person is to run out on to the road and back again without looking around until the entrails fall off. Rain water after contact with the black poplar tree was also said to be curative. Huckleberry Finn again has advice about 'spunk water' which is rainwater in a rotten tree stump. He said: 'You got to go by yourself to the middle of the woods, where you know there's a spunk water stump, and just as it's midnight you back up against the stump and jam your hand in and say: "Barley-corn, barley-corn, injun-meal shorts, spunk water, spunk water swaller these warts", and then walk away quick, eleven steps, with your eyes shut, and then turn around three times and walk home without speaking to anybody. Because if you speak the charm's busted.'[11] Other herbal remedies used in the past include bloodroot and mayapple, which both have a long history of use by Native Americans.[13] A specific recipe for wart treatments is to heat together one tablespoon of cooking salt, one tablespoon of pure saltpetre, and eight tablespoons of brandy, and enclose this in a tightly closed jar. The end of a cloth is then moistened with the mixture and the warts rubbed hard for 12 consecutive days.[8] One animal remedy once used was to have grasshoppers bite off the warts. This long-horned grasshopper (*Decticus verrucivorus*) is known in Sweden as *der Warzenbeisser* (the wart-biter).[2,12] Mineral remedies existed as wart-charming stones made of gypsum crystals that were used to rub the wart while speaking an incantation; a fee was also required.[2,10]

Miscellaneous cures have included the concepts of funerals, crossroads, knot tying, midnight, the sun or the moon, the left shoulder and odd numbers. One suggested cure from Black in 1883 was to take a small portion of earth from under the right foot at the first sight of the new moon. The earth was then made into a paste and applied on cloth to the warts. The plaster and cloth must remain on until the moon is 'out'.[6,8] Another remedy involved a stalk of rye that is cut at the time of the waning of the moon and then tied into knots equal in number to warts. This stalk was hidden for a year in a roof drain and, when the straw and knots rot away, the warts will disap-

pear. This cure would happen at the time of the waning moon. Other variations on this theme included tying knots in hair and string. In Czechoslovokia, a piece of raw meat was used to stroke the warts while a death knell sounded. While the bell tolled, the person had to speak the incantation, 'The death knell sounds I know not for whom, Your warts with him will speedily be buried. May they with him be buried'.[8] There are an endless number of ancient folk cures that are all variations on the above themes. Current alternative suggestions for wart treatment include suggestion, hypnosis and herbal treatments.[14–18] These forms of therapy may be considered by some to be the present-day version of ancient folk cures.

Although seemingly harmless, warts cause quite a lot of morbidity. They can cause social embarrassment or demoralization because they are cosmetically unacceptable to society and, therefore, to patients. Children may be teased by their friends and classmates, people have a reluctance to shake hands if a wart is present, warts can cause nail dystrophies and some people believe a wart on the nose is the mark of a witch. Warts can also cause medical problems. Painful plantar warts may lead to limping and vulvar warts can obstruct labour.[7] Warts on the fingertips of a musician can prohibit the ability to play an instrument successfully.[3] Another aspect of warts is the fear that they can cause because of their association with cancer, especially cervical cancer. For these reasons warts are just not tolerated. This also explains the multiplicity of treatment options. The problem is that viral warts are self-limiting and most will eventually disappear spontaneously, but this takes time and most people would rather face the multitude of possible harmful treatments. The wide range of folk cures and present-day cures is evidence enough to demonstrate the social impact of warts.

The impact that warts have on society can also be seen in art, music and literature. In some of his great literary works Shakespeare mentions warts. In *The Merry Wives of Windsor* Fenton has a wart above his eye about which he is curious, saying 'what of that?' in reference to the wart. Shakespeare also mentions warts in *Hamlet* when Ossa is cursed to be made 'like a wart.' *King Henry IV* makes reference to a person named Wart. Mark Twain, in *The Adventures of Tom Sawyer*, writes about folk cures for warts in a conversation between Huckleberry Finn and Tom Sawyer; they mention dead cats, spunk water and splitting a bean as cures.[11] A more recent book is *Commander Toad in Space*. This story is about a group of space adventurers who travel on a ship named Star Warts. This book makes the typical association between toads or frogs and warts. This story also makes reference to a musical called 'Warts and Peace'.[19] In 1996 a book called *Warts* was written about a girl who breaks out in warts before beginning the third grade school year. She is afraid that her school year will be ruined unless the warts go away.[20]

Warts also have an impact on movies. One of the most recent movies to make reference to warts is *Spy Kids*. Juni Cortez, one of the main characters in the movie, is a young boy afflicted by warts. In the beginning of the movie he is seen treating his warts with a bottle of clear gel medicine called wart killer. While he is putting on the medicine he says, 'Okay warts, prepare to meet your maker'. He is embarrassed to have his mother help him with treating his warts. Also, he is ridiculed at school by being called a wart hog and by being called a mummy because of the multiple bandages on his fingers. The movie makes it seem that being scared causes warts by making your hands sweat and by making you shiver. Juni's sister Carmen tells him to 'stop shaking or you'll give yourself more warts.' Another character named Floop states that sweaty hands cause warts and asks the young boy how come he has sweaty hands. Juni states that he has sweaty hands because he is scared all of the time. At the end of the

movie, this young man has outgrown his fears and suddenly finds himself free from warts.[21] Another movie that mentions warts is Monty Python's *And Now for Something Completely Different*. In this movie warts are in a song about Oliver Cromwell. The song states that Mr Cromwell is 'Lord Protector of England and his warts'.[22] It is also said that Keiko the killer whale in the movie *Free Willy* has warts.

Cinema Verité is an entire movie genre of realistic films that are supposed to show the world as it truly is. This type of realism is referred to with the phrase 'warts and all' because it is supposed to show life uncut with all the good and bad. This phrase is also used when speaking about the artistic movement of realism. Realism is said to portray life as accurately as possible, 'warts and all'.[23] Warts have also struck the Honolulu Academy of Arts. Joni Mabe's Elvis Room exhibit is a room devoted entirely to Elvis Presley. She includes in her exhibit 'The Elvis Wart'. This exhibit includes a box lined with plush red cloth that contains a test tube vial that is home to a wart from Elvis's right hand. There is also a picture showing Elvis with a wart on his right hand.[24] Mabe includes all memorabilia of Elvis, warts and all.

Warts have also found their way into a dream dictionary. This dictionary interprets what dreams mean based on the subject of the dream. It states that, 'To dream that you have a wart signifies a fall in your honor. You may also be self-punishing yourself and unwilling to forgive yourself. To dream that warts are disappearing on your hand foretells that you will overcome any obstacles to fortune. To see warts on others, signifies that you have bitter enemies nearby'.[25]

Until society removes the stigma attached to warts, individual people will not be able to live with their warts free of shame. Maybe more people should try to accept these little growths. We should look to Oliver Cromwell for advice. He said to Sir Peter Lely, 'I desire you would use all your skill to paint my picture truly like me and not flatter me at all; but remark all these roughnesses, pimples, warts, and everything as you see me, otherwise I will not pay a farthing for it'.[5,11]

REFERENCES

1. Lempiere WW. Treatment of warts. *Aust J Dermatol* 1951; **1**: 34–7.
2. Burns DA. 'Warts and all' – the history and folklore of warts: a review. *J R Soc Med* 1992; **85**: 37–40.
3. Bunney MH. Warts through the ages: from mythology to virology. In: *Viral Warts: their biology and treatment*. Oxford: Oxford University Press, 1982: 5–9.
4. Birley HD. Continuing medical ignorance: modern myths in the management of genital warts. *Int J STD AIDS* 2001; **12**: 71–4.
5. Bett WR. 'Wart, I bid thee begone.' *Practitioner* 1951; **166**: 77–80.
6. Rolleston JD. Dermatology and folk-lore. *Br J Dermatol* 1940; **52**: 43–57.
7. Doorbar J. Warts and all. *Mill Hill Essays from National Institute for Medical Research* 1999 http://www.nimr.mrc.ac.uk/MillHillEssays/ 1999/warts.html.
8. Ross MS. Warts in the medical folklore of Europe. *Int J Dermatol* 1979; **18**: 505–9.
9. Trevelyan M. Folk-lore and folk-stories of Wales: charms, pentacles and spells. *V Wales* 2002. http://www.red4.co.uk/folklore/trevelyan/ welshfolklore/chapt17.htm
10. Roberts N. Wart charming stone. *J R Coll Gen Pract* 1988; **38**: 93.
11. Twain M. *The Adventures of Tom Sawyer*. New York: Harper Bros, c1938.
12. Bleiberg J. Witchcraft, warts and wisdom. *J Med Soc New Jersey* 1957; **54**: 123–6.
13. Tucker AO. Herbal remedies for warts. *Herbs for Health* 1999; **00**: 51–3.
14. Dreaper R. Recalcitrant warts on the hand cured by hypnosis. *Practitioner* 1978; **220**: 305–10.
15. Gravitz MA. The production of warts by suggestion as a cultural phenomenon. *Am J Clin Hypnosis* 1981; **23**: 281–2.
16. Harper J. Warts: the holistic health centre. *Here's Health* 2001; March: 45.
17. Spanos NP, Williams V, Gwynn MI. Effects of hypnotic, placebo and salicylic acid treatments on wart regression. *Psychosom Med* 1990; **52**: 109–14.
18. Straatmeyer AJ, Rhodes NR. Condyloma acuminata: Results of treatment using hypnosis. *J Am Acad Dermatol* 1983; **9**: 434–6.
19. Yolen J. *Commander Toad in Space*. New York: Coward, McCann & Geoghegan, 1980.
20. Shreve S. *Warts*. Tambourine books, 1996.
21. Rodriguez, Robert. *Spy Kids*. Dimension Films & Troublemaker Studios, 2001.
22. Monty Python Song Lyrics, 'Oliver Cromwell'. http://www.stone-dead.asn.au/ albums-cds/lyrics/oliver-cromwell.htm
23. McConnell R. *French Realism & Cinema Verite*. Robert McConnell Productions, 1999. http://www.parlez-vous.com/misc/realism.htm
24. Memminger C. *Elvis Lives at Academy of Warts, er, Arts*. Honolulu Lite: Honolulu Star-Bulletin, 1997. http://www.starbulletin.com/ lite/elvis.htm.
25. Dream Dictionary. http://www.dreammoods. com/dreamdictionary/w.htm

2 Papillomaviruses: biology and analysis

Walter G Hubert

Viral structure and classification • Genetic functions • Viral life cycle and molecular pathogenesis • Host immune response • Analytical methods • Outlook • References

Papillomaviruses (PVs) are small DNA viruses that infect numerous vertebrate hosts, including humans. Viral infection targets epithelial cells and progeny virions are produced upon cellular differentiation. Although infection with most of the 85 human viral types identified to date leads to benign hyperproliferative lesions or warts,[1] typically on the extremities, a small number of human PVs (HPVs) are causally associated with the development of anogenital cancer. Such oncogenic HPVs include types 16, 18, 31, 33 and 35, and are referred to as high-risk viruses to indicate the high probability for malignant progression after infection.[2] Other HPVs associated with human neoplasia are epidermodysplasia verruciformis (EV)-inducing types. This rare form of skin cancer may result from infection with HPV types 5 or 8 if the host has a genetic predisposition for EV. All PVs infect keratinocytes, and are believed to initiate infection through microscopic lacerations in the epithelium, which provides access to basal cells. Only the fibropapillomaviruses of ungulate animals can infect dermal fibroblasts as well as epithelial host cells. HPVs exhibit a high degree of tissue tropism and specific viral types infect either the cutaneous epithelium or the oral/genital mucosa. All PVs are disseminated by direct contact and genital HPVs are usually transmitted sexually.[3] HPV epidemiology is described in Chapter 3 and the clinical manifestations of viral infections in Chapter 4.

This chapter first provides an introduction to the biology of HPVs, including their classification, genetic functions, viral life cycle and pathogenesis, and goes on to describe the common methods used to analyse HPV infections and biology in the clinical and research laboratory settings. Table 2.1 is a list of the abbreviations covering this subject.

VIRAL STRUCTURE AND CLASSIFICATION

Virus structure and families

As a result of their virion stucture, PVs are grouped together with the slightly smaller polyomaviruses (PyVs), which include polyoma and vacuolating virus types, such as murine PyV and simian virus 40 (SV40), respectively.[4] The name of the Papovavirus family is derived from the representing families of *pa*pilloma, *po*lyoma and *va*cuolating viruses.[3] HPV capsids, such as those of other Papovavirinae, are icosahedral, and display two-, three- and fivefold centres of symmetry. Their capsid structure of $T = 7$ requires that the 72 capsomers are arranged in a sphere, with each

Table 2.1 Abbreviations

Item	Meaning	Item	Meaning
AdV	adenovirus	HPV	human papillomavirus
AE	auxilliary enhancer	IFN	interferon
AP1	activator protein 1	ISGF	interferon-stimulated gene factor
AT	adenine–thymine	Jak	Janus kinase
ATP	adenosine triphosphate	kDa	kilodalton
bp	base-pair	KE	keratinocyte enhancer
BPV	bovine papillomavirus	LCR	long control region
CBP	CAMP responsive element binding protein binding protein	LT	large tumour antigen
		Mcm	multicopy maintenance protein
CDP	CCAAT displacement protein	Oct	octamer-binding protein
CEBP	CAAT enhancer-binding protein	ORF	translational open reading frame
CIN	cervical intraepithelial neoplasia	PCPV	pygmy chimpanzee papillomavirus
CKI	cyclin-dependent kinase inhibitor	PCR	polymerase chain reaction
COPV	canine oral papillomavirus	PV	papillomavirus
CRPV	cotton-tail rabbit papillomavirus	PyV	polyomavirus
DPV	deer papillomavirus	Rb	retinoblastoma protein
E6AP	E6-associated protein	RhPV	rhesus monkey papillomavirus
E6BP	E6-binding protein	RT	reverse transcription
E6TP	E6-targeted protein	Sp1	specificity factor
EGF	epidermal growth factor	STAT	signal transducer and activator of transcription
ERC-55	endoplasmic reticulum calcium-binding protein 55 kDa		
		SV40	simian virus 40
EV	epidermodysplasia verruciformis	TBP	TATA box-binding protein
Fp1	footprint 1	TEF	transcription-enhancing factor
H1, H4	core histone 1 and 4	Tyk	tyrosine kinase
HDAC	histone deacetylase	URR	upstream regulatory region
hDlg	human homologue of drosophila disc large protein	UTR	untranslated region
		YY	yin yang factor

capsomer having either five or six neighbours. PV virions are non-enveloped, and have a capsid diameter of 55–60 nm, made up entirely of viral proteins.[5] The viral genome of about 8000 base-pairs (bp) is carried within the capsid as a mini-chromosome, where the circular viral DNA is associated with host-derived core histones (H1–H4).

Functionally, PVs belong to the small DNA tumour virus family which also includes PyVs and adenoviruses (AdVs). This classification is based on the common strategies of these viruses to regulate cellular processes. In particular, the E7 protein from high-risk HPVs, the large tumour (LT) antigen of SV40 and the E1A protein of human AdV have protein domains in common, which are required for binding to the cell cycle-regulatory pocket proteins (p105 Rb, p107, p130).[6,7] Furthermore, E6 from high-risk HPVs, SV40-LT and AdV-E1B also have binding domains specific for the p53 tumour suppressor protein.[8,9]

Table 2.2 Common HPV types and induced diseases

Primary site of infection	HPV type	Disease
Cutaneous skin, extremities	1, 2, 27	Warts
	5, 8	Epidermodysplasia verruciformis
Oral mucosa	11	Juvenile laryngeal papillomatosis
External genital mucosa	6, 11	Condyloma acuminata
Internal genital mucosa	16, 18, 31, 33	Cervical intraepithelial neoplasia, cervical cancer

Papillomavirus nomenclature

Unlike serotypes with AdVs, PVs are organized by host and genotype. Among the vertebrate hosts are the cotton-tail rabbit (CRPV), cattle (bovine, BPV), deer (DPV), dogs (canine oral, COPV), rhesus monkey (RhPV), pygmy chimpanzee (PCPV) and humans (HPV). The viruses within each host group are numbered in the order of their discovery. New genotypes must have at least a 10% difference in the nucleotide sequences of the upstream regulatory region (URR), E6 (early) and L2 (late) genes when compared with known PVs. Sequence differences between 2% and 10% are classified as subtypes and less than 2% as variants of a given viral type.[10] For epidemiological purposes, HPVs are commonly grouped by pathogenesis and tissue tropism. Among the cutaneous HPVs, there are non-oncogenic types that cause common warts as well as oncogenic, EV-associated ones. Mucosal HPVs are referred to as either low-risk viruses, which include the types that induce benign oral or genital infections, or high-risk viruses which are associated with malignant genital lesions.[3] Table 2.2 contains an abridged overview of the most commonly found HPV types, their tissue tropism and the associated diseases.

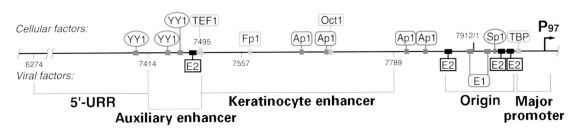

Figure 2.1
Upstream regulatory region (URR) of HPV31: this schematic representation of the URR shows the position of the DNA-binding sites for cellular (above) and viral (below) proteins that participate in the regulation of HPV gene expression and DNA replication. The functional domains are also indicated: 5'-URR, auxilliary enhancer (AE), keratinocyte enhancer (KE), replication origin (Ori), major promoter (P_{97}) region. Nucleotide positions in the HPV31 genome refer to the published sequence.[11]

GENETIC FUNCTIONS

Genomic organization

The genomes of all known PVs are organized in a similar fashion and include common, translational, open reading frames (ORFs).[3] A non-coding, URR, also called the long control region or LCR, contains binding sites for transcription factors as well as an origin of DNA replication (Figure 2.1). Other *cis*-regulatory elements, such as promoters, polyadenylation signals and mRNA splicing sites that act only on the viral DNA molecule on which they reside, are found throughout the viral genome (Figure 2.2). The typical PV genome encodes up to 10 genes in overlapping ORFs, which are transcribed unidirectionally and grouped into either early or late regions (Figure 2.2). The viral proteins encoded by these genes function in *trans*, i.e. they are diffusible and can act on all viral genomes or specific host proteins within a cell. Early genes are expressed throughout the viral life cycle whereas late genes only in differentiated keratinocytes. Most of the HPV-encoded genes can be placed into three functional groups: regulatory proteins that primarily control viral processes

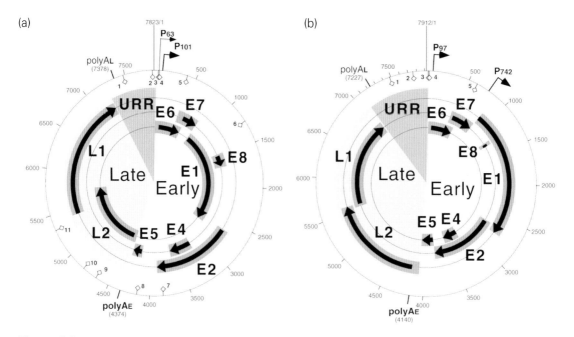

Figure 2.2
Genomic maps of HPV types (a) 27 (cutaneous) and (b) 31 (mucosal): the organization of HPV genomes is conserved: early and late regions as well as the upstream regulatory region (URR). Viral transcription is unidirectional and occurs from promoters in the early region (arrows at the periphery). Translational open reading frames (stippled arcs) contain early (E) and late (L) genes (solid arcs with arrows). Viral messenger RNAs are polyadenylated at signals downstream of the respective protein-coding sequences, poly$_{AE}$ and poly$_{AL}$. The E2 DNA-binding sites in the viral genomes are shown at the periphery (numbered diamond flags).

Table 2.3 *cis*-Acting elements on the HPV genome

Element	Functions	Factor-binding sites
Upstream regulatory region		
5'-URR	Late polyadenylation signal	
	Transcriptional silencer	CDP
Auxilliary enhancer	Conditional transcriptional enhancer	E2, YY1, TEF1
Keratinocyte enhancer	Cell-specific transcriptional enhancer	AP1, Oct1
	Replication enhancer	
Replication origin	Initiation of viral DNA synthesis	E1 and E2
P_{97} promoter	Transcriptional start for early mRNAs	TBP
Early region		
E6 intron	mRNA splicing for E7 mRNA	
P_{742} promoter	Transcriptional start for late mRNAs	
E1–E4 intron	mRNA splicing for E1–E4 protein	
E8–E2 intron	mRNA splicing for E8–E2C repressor	
3'-UTR	Early polyadenylation signal	
Late region		
E2–L1 intron	mRNA splicing for L1 protein	

See Table 2.1 for abbreviations.

(transcription and replication); regulatory proteins that modulate cellular processes (proliferation, differentiation, apoptosis); and the structural virion components.[12] The major *cis*-acting elements of the HPV genome, as well as the viral proteins and their functions, are described below and listed in Tables 2.3 and 2.4, respectively.

cis-Regulatory elements

The URR of HPVs, as exemplified by that of the high-risk HPV31 (see Figure 2.1), contains multiple functional domains: a 5'-region (5'-URR), a conditional (auxiliary) transcriptional enhancer (AE),[13] a cell-specific (keratinocyte) enhancer (KE),[14] the replication origin and a major viral promoter (P_{101} in HPV27, P_{97} in

HPV31 – Figure 2.2). The function of the 5'-domain of the URR is not well characterized but it is known to repress viral transcription and DNA replication of some HPV types moderately.[15,16] The AE of HPVs contains binding sites for E2 and cellular transcription factors, activates the major viral promoter at low levels of E2,[17] and is required for viral DNA replication.[16] Viral gene expression is primarily regulated by cellular transcription factors, which bind to the KE and modulate the activity of the major viral promoter. Although many of the factor binding sites have already been identified in this enhancer element of HPV31 (AP1, Oct1, etc.), others remain to be characterized (foot print 1 or Fp1). AE- and KE-mediated transcriptional regulation depends on the abundance, as well as the different activities, of the cellular transcription factors. In the case of AP1, which is one of the major

Table 2.4 *trans*-Acting functions of HPVs

Gene(s)	Group	Function
Early region		
E6 (high-risk)	Oncogene	Binding to and degradation of p53
		Induction of telomerase
		'Anti-apoptotic'
E7 (high-risk)	Oncogene	Binding to retinoblastoma protein, release of E2F
		'Mitogenic'
E1	Replication factor	ATP-dependent DNA helicase
E1–E4	Unknown	May assist in viral egress
E8–E2C	Transcription factor	Repressor
E2	Transcription factor	Activator of P_{97} at low levels
		Repression of P_{97} at high levels
	Replication factor	Positioning of E1/E2 initiation complex
E5	Oncogene	Activation of cellular growth factor receptors
Late region		
L2	Capsid protein	Minor structural protein
L1	Capsid protein	Major structural protein

activators in HPV31,[14] transcriptional regulation is also accomplished by subunit mixing of multiple Jun and Fos proteins as a function of cellular differentiation. The origin is required for viral DNA replication and contains DNA-binding sites for the viral replication factors E1 and E2, as well as an AT-rich region within the palindromic E1 site[18] (see Figure 2.1).

The major viral promoter (P_{97} for HPV16 and 31) contains a consensus TATA box and is located at the 3' boundary of the URR. P_{97} is strongly activated by the KE and, to a lesser degree, by the AE.[13,14] This promoter is active throughout the viral life cycle and its mRNAs encode E6, E7, E1, E2 and E5. Early viral mRNAs are polyadenylated at the early polyAE signal located in the 3'-untranslated region (UTR), downstream of E5 (see Figure 2.2). The structure of the differentiation-specific promoter (P_{742} in HPV31) is similar to that of a cellular housekeeping promoter, in that it does not contain a consensus TATA box. In addition, no proximal binding sites for cellular transcription factors have been identified for P_{742}. This promoter is active during vegetative viral DNA replication and produces mRNAs for E1, E1–E4, L2 and L1. These late mRNAs are polyadenylated at the late polyAL signal located 3' to the L1 gene (see Figure 2.2). The regulation of viral gene expression is complex and, aside from different promoters, is modulated significantly by mRNA splicing (reviewed in Lamains[12]). Numerous splicing signals can be found throughout the early and late regions of the viral genome. Most notable in high-risk HPVs is the E6 intron which is involved in regulating E7 and E1. Expression of the transcriptional repressor E8–E2C, the E1–E4 protein and the structural L1 proteins also involves the removal of specific introns from the viral mRNAs, which are mostly polycistronic.

Virus-directed regulatory proteins

The HPV functions that regulate viral gene expression and plasmid replication are E1 and E2.[19] Both proteins bind to DNA and recognize sites within the URR, replication origin, major promoter region, and other regions of the viral genome (see Figures 2.1 and 2.2). E1 is the largest and most conserved protein among all PVs. It is an ATP-dependent DNA helicase and functions in HPV DNA replication, in an analogous way to SV40-LT. Before the initiation of viral DNA synthesis, E1 and E2 form a multimeric protein complex at the replication origin, which recruits the cellular proteins required for DNA synthesis, such as primase, DNA polymerase and replication protein A.[20,21] E2 is a multifunctional protein that regulates viral transcription and DNA replication. It binds DNA with high affinity at palindromic recognition sites that have an $ACC(H_6)GGT$ structure.[22] At low protein levels, E2 activates transcription from the major viral promoter by binding to its site 1, located in the AE (see Figure 2.1). At high protein levels, E2 can repress viral transcription from the major promoter by binding to sites 3 and 4, which are located adjacent to the promoter's TATA box.[17] In high-risk HPVs, an additional form of E2-mediated regulation involves an E8–E2C fusion protein which is translated from a spliced mRNA and contains several amino acids from the E8 gene and the C-terminal half of the E2. E8–E2C lacks the N-terminal transactivation domain of E2 and, therefore, represses E2-mediated viral transcription and DNA replication.[23]

Host-directed regulatory proteins

All PVs encode three oncogenes: E6, E7 and E5. E6 and E7 are the major oncogenes of high-risk mucosal HPVs, and E5 plays a less established role in viral pathogenesis. The functions of the viral oncogenes in low-risk mucosal and cutaneous HPVs are not well characterized. However, as is the case with high-risk HPVs, these genes are implicated in the regulation of cell growth and differentiation during the life cycle of the non-oncogenic HPV types.

Numerous cellular proteins have been identified that interact with E7 from high-risk HPVs. These include: the pocket proteins p105 retinoblastoma (Rb[7]), p107[24] and p130;[24] the cyclins A[24,25] and E;[26] cyclin-dependent kinase inhibitors (CKI) p21[27,28] and p27;[29] histone H1 kinase;[30] histone deacetylase (HDAC) 1;[31] members of the AP1 family of transcription factors;[32] and the interferon-stimulated gene factor ISGF3γ. Binding of these cellular regulators to high-risk E7 promotes cell-cycle progression by transcriptionally activating S-phase-specific genes and inactivating the G1 and G2/mitotic spindle checkpoints. Other biological functions of high-risk E7 include the inhibition of cell cycle exit, retention of nuclei in differentiated suprabasal cells and induction of apoptosis. Finally, high-risk E7 also diminishes interferon-α-mediated signalling through the signal transducer and activator of transcription (STAT) 1 pathway. Although the E7 proteins from high- and low-risk HPVs can be distinguished by differences in their binding affinities to pocket proteins, which is high only with high-risk E7 proteins,[33] all E7 proteins associate with CKIs to regulate cell growth. As low-risk E7 proteins do not bind strongly to Rb family members, low-risk HPVs are not able to immortalize primary keratinocytes. Nevertheless, low-risk E7 can overcome the p21- and p27-mediated checkpoint in the G1 phase.[34] Therefore, the induction of efficient cellular proliferation observed after infection with cutaneous or low-risk mucosal HPV may in part be controlled through the same molecular mechanisms that high-risk HPVs utilize.

Expression of high-risk E6 proteins results in the transformation of fibroblasts, immortalization of keratinocytes and transcriptional modulation of heterologous promoters in transient assays. At present, the mechanisms of transcriptional regulation by E6 are not known and this activity of E6 does not correlate with its known transforming/immortalizing functions (reviewed in Rapp and Chen[35]). Numerous cellular proteins have been identified that bind to E6 and the biological functions of these interactions are well characterized. E6 can bind to the tumour suppressor p53,[8] the E6-associated protein (E6AP or ubiquitin ligase E3[36]), the replication licensing factor multi-copy maintenance (Mcm) protein 7,[37,38] the transcriptional coactivator CBP/p300,[39,40] the human homologue of the drosophila Disc Large tumour suppressor protein (hDlg[41,42]), a putative GTPase-activating protein E6TP1 (E6-targeted protein 1[43]), the calcium-binding protein ERC-55 (also termed E6-binding protein or E6BP[44]), the focal adhesion protein paxillin,[45] the clathrin-adaptor AP-1,[46] the interferon regulatory factor (IRF) 3,[47] and the cytoplasmic tyrosine kinase Tyk2.[48] The interactions of E6 with these cellular regulators lead to E6/E6AP-induced degradation of p53, inactivation of the G1 cell cycle checkpoint, abrogation of the G2/mitotic spindle checkpoint, induction of telomerase during cellular immortalization, as well as E6-mediated prevention of apoptosis and resistance to differentiation. Additional cellular proteins bind to E6 and are implicated in p53-independent transformation of cells. E6 can also modulate interferon signalling by multiple mechanisms. E6 proteins from low-risk and high-risk HPVs have some common cellular binding partners but differ in their ability to immortalize or transform cells. Low-risk E6 also activates transcription from viral promoters but its significance in HPV-mediated pathogenesis is not known.[35]

E5 is the major oncogene in fibropapillomaviruses such as BPV1, but the role of E5 in the pathogenesis of HPVs is much less clear. As with fibropapillomaviruses, E5 from high-risk HPVs is known to interact with a subunit of the pore-forming vacuolar ATPase.[49,50] High-risk E5 also increases tyrosine phosphorylation of the EGF receptor, and inhibits turnover of this receptor.[51] Interestingly, E5 proteins from cutaneous HPVs appear to be more closely related to BPV E5 than E5 proteins from mucosal HPVs.[52]

Although E4 is the most abundantly expressed viral protein,[53] its biological role in the viral life cycle has not been fully established. In the high-risk HPV types 16 and 31, it is an E1–E4 fusion protein and, despite its location in the early region of the viral genome, it is expressed only as a late protein in the terminal layers of the epithelium. E1–E4 of HPV16 has been found to affect the cyctoskeletal structure by interfering with actin filament assembly and, therefore, may aid viral egress.[54]

Structural proteins

HPV virions contain only a major and a minor structural protein, L1 and L2 respectively. Once expressed in suprabasal keratinocytes, L1 spontaneously aggregates into pentameric capsomers[55] which make up most of the protein content of the viral capsid. The function of L2 in viral encapsidation has not been elucidated conclusively, although it is known to localize to distinct nuclear domains during virion assembly[56] and may also aid in viral uptake during the initiation of infection.[57]

VIRAL LIFE CYCLE AND MOLECULAR PATHOGENESIS

The molecular events during pathogenesis have been studied most conclusively with high-risk HPVs. Nevertheless, the basic descriptions of the individual phases of the viral life cycle apply to all HPVs. From the perspective of pathogenesis, the viral life cyle can be divided into two stages (Figure 2.3):

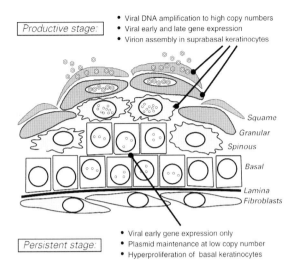

Productive stage:
- Viral DNA amplification to high copy numbers
- Viral early and late gene expression
- Virion assembly in suprabasal keratinocytes

Squame
Granular
Spinous
Basal
Lamina
Fibroblasts

Persistent stage:
- Viral early gene expression only
- Plasmid maintenance at low copy number
- Hyperproliferation of basal keratinocytes

Figure 2.3
Cross-section of a wart: this schematic representation of a cutaneous wart shows the HPV life cycle. During the persistent stage, HPV virions infect the basal cells, express early viral genes and establish a low plasmid copy number that is maintained in an expanding basal cell population. The productive stage of HPV infection requires cellular differentiation (spinous, granular cells). Viral DNA copy number is amplified, late genes are expressed, and progeny virions assembled and shed.

(1) during the persistent stage, HPV DNA can be found in the basal cell population for several months to many years. This stage is characterized by low levels of viral replication and stable inheritance of HPV DNA by daughter cells for many cell generations. (2) The productive stage of the life cycle takes place only in terminally differentiated, suprabasal keratinocytes, and involves vegetative viral DNA amplification, capsid gene expression and virion assembly. At the molecular level, the PV life cycle is divided into three phases of viral DNA replication: establishment, maintenance and DNA amplification (reviewed in Howley[3]) which are described below in greater detail.

HPV establishment

Virions of HPV infect the basal epithelium after gaining access through microscopic lacerations. The mechanism of viral uptake is not well understood, however, both the $\alpha6/\beta4$ integrin-complex and the heparan-containing proteoglycans have been implicated as viral receptors.[58–60] After transport to the nucleus, expression of the early viral genes commences. Over the course of several cell generations, the infecting HPV DNA establishes itself as an autonomously replicating, low copy number plasmid of 25–50 per cell.[61] The increase of viral copy number from as few as one infectious virion[62] to this optimal copy number requires that the viral DNA replicates more frequently than once per cell cycle. During the establishment phase, the early gene products of E1 and E2 mediate viral transcription and DNA replication whereas E6 and E7 increase the fraction of proliferating cells within the basal keratinocyte population.

HPV maintenance

The persistent phase of the viral life cycle is characterized by expression of the viral early genes and stable plasmid replication. As a consequence of the anti-apoptotic and mitogenic activities of E6 and E7, respectively, the HPV-positive basal cell population is expanded. Continual cellular proliferation and limited differentiation provide an environment that is conducive for stable replication. During this phase, the viral copy number is maintained at 25–50 per cell for many cell generations through E1– and E2-modulated viral transcription and DNA replication. On average, the viral genomes replicate once per cell cycle during maintenance.[63] Although the molecular details that affect the length of viral persistence are not known, it is expected that it is strongly affected by the host's immune response.

HPV DNA amplification

When HPV-positive basal keratinocytes begin to differentiate, the viral copy number increases to several thousand in a subset of these cells. During this phase of the viral life cycle, the viral oncogenes are involved in preventing enucleation of HPV-infected keratinocytes, which would normally occur in differentiating epithelial cells. The differentiated HPV-positive keratinocytes therefore retain the capacity to replicate viral DNA and express the structural viral proteins. The process of vegetative viral DNA replication, which is mediated by E1 and E2, may be similar to an extended S phase of the cell cycle. Amplification of viral DNA is a prerequisite for the expression of the late or stuctural viral genes in the terminal layers of the epithelium.[61] The L1 and L2 proteins assemble into viral capsomers and the HPV DNA is packaged into the capsid as a mini-chromosome. HPV virions are infectious and do not require further maturation steps such as proteolytic cleavage of capsid proteins. Viral progeny particles are shed with the squames from the surface of the epithelium to begin a new infectious cycle.

PV-mediated induction of malignancy

During the normal life cycle when the DNA of oncogenic HPVs replicates as a plasmid, E6 and E7 are expressed under viral control, leading to a moderate level of oncoproteins in cells. Viral control of early gene expression involves the activation of the major viral promoter by the KE in the URR and dose-dependent repression by the E2 protein. The continual presence of low levels of viral oncoproteins through many cell generations can induce genetic instability in HPV-infected cells. As a consequence, such cells may aquire other genetic changes over time, and also

integrate the viral DNA into the cellular genome, as is frequently observed with HPV16.[12] Integration of the HPV DNA places E6 and E7 expression primarily under cellular control, which elevates the steady-state levels of the viral oncoproteins[64] and provides such cells with a higher proliferative capacity.[65] Two distinct mechanisms account for this increase in E6/E7 expression: (1) integration typically disrupts the E2 protein coding sequence;[66] (2) E6/E7 mRNAs from integrated HPV DNA contain a new cellular 3'-untranslated region which reduces their turnover rate in vivo.[67] Integration of HPV DNA into the cellular chromosome is not, however, strictly required for tumorigenesis because autonomously replicating viral DNA can be found in HPV16-, 18- and 31-induced tumors.

HOST IMMUNE RESPONSE

Infection by HPVs elicits unique antiviral, humoral and cellular immune responses from the host. Although our understanding of the role that these host responses play in HPV pathogenesis is still limited, tremendous strides in understanding HPV-related immunology have been made in the past few years. Several aspects of the host immune response to HPV infection will also be presented in Chapters 13, 15 and 17.

Cellular antiviral response

The capacity of high-risk HPVs to modulate the host immune responses has recently been analysed. Interferons (IFNs) are cytokines that regulate cellular proliferation and also modulate the immune response to viral infection (reviewed in Vilcek and Sen[68]). The known IFN types α, β and γ use the Jak-STAT pathway of signal transduction to activate IFN-responsive genes.[69] The expression of IFNα and IFNβ is transcriptionally regulated by the interferon regulatory factors (IRFs). Recent in vitro studies have shown that high-risk E7 can bind to ISGF3γ, a protein in the STAT family, and therefore inhibit the activation of IFNα-responsive genes,[70,71] reducing signalling. In addition to the downregulation by E7, high-risk E6 can modulate the interferon response by two independent mechanisms. First, E6 can bind to IRF3 and thus diminish IFNβ expression.[47] Second, IFNα-mediated signalling is downregulated when E6 binds to Tyk2 kinase to prevent its autophosphorylation and phosphorylation of the STAT proteins. The multiple interactions of E6 and E7 with proteins involved in the IFNα and IFNβ signaling cascades thus contribute to the overall down-modulation of the cellular antiviral responses without affecting the IFNγ pathway.[48,72] The oncoprotein-mediated suppression of the IFNα pathway may in part account for the poor success rate of IFNα therapy against high-risk HPV infections.[73]

Cellular and humoral response

The cellular immune response after HPV infection is complex and involves the induction of cellular adhesion molecules, altered cytokine production and changes in expression of major histocompatibility complex (MHC) molecules. These HPV-induced changes are believed to contribute to the creation of a local zone of immune cell depletion which surrounds the site of infection (reviewed in Tyring[10]). It is also known that 35–60% of HPV-infected individuals have low titres of capsid-specific antibodies.[74]

Vaccine development

Our increased knowledge about the host's immune response to HPV infection provides the basis for the development of prophylactic and therapeutic vaccines.

This is currently a very active area of HPV-related research, in which animal models and early human trials are used to assess the efficacy of vaccines in eliciting protective antibodes and cytotoxic T-cell responses (reviewed in Da Silva et al[75]). HPV-specific vaccines are developed with peptide domains from HPV proteins, entire viral proteins, virus-like particles (empty capsids), and either DNA vectors or recombinant viral vectors encoding HPV genes.

ANALYTICAL METHODS

Methods for the clinical laboratory

The analytical methods used in the clinical laboratory must accomplish high sensitivity and accuracy in a manageable assay format. As the severity of HPV-mediated disease is strongly dependent on the viral type, assays to detect HPV in clinical biopsies must also identify the viral type for accurate prognosis. The following methods have been developed primarily for the analysis of genital HPV infections, because the risk for malignant disease is much greater with these viral types than with cutaneous ones.

Cytology

This is still the most commonly employed method for analysing HPV-induced lesions because most clinical laboratories are set up to perform fixation,[76] sectioning[77] and staining of tissue samples. In the case of suspected infections with genital HPVs, exfoliated cells from the uterine cervix are usually analysed by the

Papanicolaou (Pap) smear test. This diagnostic method has been a significant factor in reducing the incidence of cervical intraepithelial neoplasia (CIN) and the more advanced malignancies in countries where regular screening is available.[78] Today, with the help of computerized sample processing, the accuracy of this test for the detection of atypical cells has been increased even further.[79] The major limitation of the Pap smear and other cytological methods is the fact that they cannot determine the type of HPV present in the biopsy specimen. Type-specific identification of HPV DNA in clinical samples can be accomplished by several newer assays described below.

Hybrid-capture assay

This analytical method was developed to provide fast, sensitive and type-specific detection of HPV DNA with minimal requirements for technical equipment.[80] It is used primarily for the detection of mucosal HPV types in oral and genital infections, and is based on the specific interaction of viral RNA probes in a reaction mixture with complementary HPV DNA present in biopsy samples (Figure 2.4). After viral RNA–DNA hybrids form they can be immobilized with a hybrid-specific antibody. The immobilized hybrids are subsequently detected with a second antibody which is conjugated to alkaline phosphatase. The sample is then analysed by chemiluminescence in a luminometer to measure the amount of emitted light.

Polymerase chain reaction-mediated detection and typing

Lesions containing HPV, in general, exhibit a low abundance of most viral regulatory proteins. In benign infections, only the major

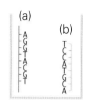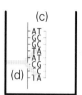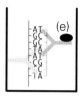

Figure 2.4
Hybrid-capture assay: this standardized assay system is used in conjunction with colposcopy and Pap smear analysis of cervical lesions. (a) Preparation: the DNA in biopsy samples is denatured to form single-stranded targets in solution. (b) Probing: RNA probe mixtures are added. (c) Hybridization: specific RNA–DNA hybrids form if the correct target sequences are present. (d) Immobilization: samples are transfered to a new tube precoated with antibodies that recognize RNA–DNA hybrids. The hybrids are retained during washes. (e) Detection: the presence of RNA–DNA hybrids is detected with a second, enzyme-conjugated antibody, and visualized by chemiluminescence.

capsid protein L1 or the E4 protein can usually be detected in the suprabasal cell layers.[81] In high-risk HPV infections, particularly during the advanced stages of malignant disease, the viral DNA is often integrated into the cellular genome and only the oncoproteins E6 and E7 are expressed. Therefore, the most reliable indicator of HPV infection is the presence of viral DNA. For this reason, a polymerase chain reaction (PCR) type of assay is the method of choice for sensitive detection and reliable typing of HPVs.

PCR is based on the amplification of target DNA which can be present at very low concentrations in the clinical sample.[82] Repeated cycles of denaturing (separating strands) the target and product DNAs at high temperature (95°C), annealing (binding) of complementary oligo-DNA primers to sites within the template (original target and new DNA strands) at a low

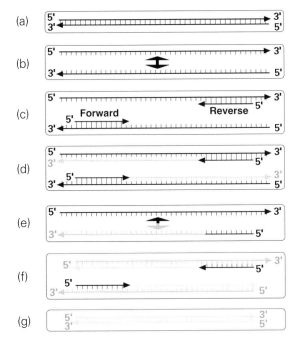

Figure 2.5
Principles of the polymerase chain reaction
(PCR): PCR is a versatile and sensitive method
for HPV detection and typing in both the clinical
and the research laboratory. (a) Preparation:
purified sample DNA serves as template in a
reaction mixture which contains a thermostable
DNA polymerase, a pair of forward and reverse
oligo-DNA primers, deoxyribonucleotides and
buffer. (b) In a thermocycler, the template DNA
is denatured at high temperature for several
minutes at the start of the PCR programme. (c)
The temperature is lowered to a point that
favours the specific annealing of primers to
their target sequences on both strands of the
DNA template. (d) New DNA strands of
indefinite length are synthesized by the
polymerase beginning at the 3'-termini of the
annealed primers when the temperature is
raised moderately. (e) Template and new
daughter strands are denatured again at high
temperature. (f) Primers are annealed again to
begin the second cycle. The previously
synthesized strands now act as templates of
defined length. (g) Thermal cycling is repeated
25–35 times, during which the abundance of a
PCR product of defined size is amplified
geometrically.

temperature (50–65°C), and then extending
(synthesizing) new DNA daughter strands from
these primers at an intermediate temperature
(75°C), are applied to amplify the concentration
of the target sequences geometrically (Figure
2.5). This process is performed automatically in
a programmable thermal cycler, using heat-
stable DNA polymerases such as Taq (isolated
originally from *Thermus aquaticus*).

As practically all known HPVs can be
detected with high sensitivity and typed,[83–85]
PCR can provide accurate and fast diagnosis of
lesions presumed to be HPV positive. For this
purpose, successive PCR reactions are
performed with the same biopsy sample first
to identify the HPV class (cutaneous, mucosal),
and then to identify the group (phylogenetically
related types) and, finally if desired, the individual viral type[86] (Figure 2.6). Class- and group-
specific primer pairs are degenerate, i.e. they
recognize multiple HPV types, whereas type-
specific primers bind to only one viral type.

Southern blotting

This method was the earliest way of detecting
and typing HPVs in DNA isolated from
biopsies. It is still widely used in both clinical
and research laboratories, often in conjunction
with PCR-based amplification of viral DNA. The
versatility of Southern blotting does not come
only from its high sensitivity; it also permits an
analysis of the replicative state of the HPV
DNA in infected cells. Different topological
forms of the HPV DNA, either integrated (non-
replicating) or relaxed and closed circular (both
indicating replicating HPV) can be identified.
Similarly, viral DNA fragments of different size
can be resolved, which provides a fingerprint
of a given HPV type when sample DNA is
digested with appropriate restriction enzymes.
The principle of detection in Southern blot
assays is based on the specific hybridization of
complementary DNA or RNA probes to sample

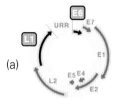

(a)

(b) HVP2: 5'-d(TCNMGNGGNCANCCNYTNGG)

(c) CN3F: 5'-d(AACTCTAAYATWGCACATG)

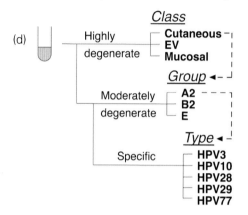

(d)

Figure 2.6
PCR-mediated HPV typing: using PCR, biopsies can quickly be screened for the presence of specific HPV types to facilitate accurate risk assessment for the patient. (a) Degenerate primer locations: L1 and E6 are relatively conserved genes among all papillomaviruses and degenerate primer sites, allowing for the detection of multiple HPV types located in these coding sequences. (b) Example of a highly degenerate primer that recognizes the entire cutaneous HPV class.[86] Degeneracy is high as a result of the numerous N (any nucleotide), M (A or C) and Y (T or C). (c) Example of a moderately degenerate primer that is specific for the cutaneous HPV group A2.[86] Degeneracy is low because of only one Y (T or C) and one W (A or T). (d) Typing scheme: in separate PCR reactions using the same biopsy DNAs template, the HPV class is determined first, then the group and, finally, the individual HPV type. (EV, epidermodysplasia verruciformis.)

DNA.[87] Such probes can be generated from known HPV DNA by labelling with nucleotides that contain radioisotopes (^{32}P, ^{35}S), fluorophores (fluorescein) or a molecular tag (digoxigenin, avidin) for detection.

Typically, the purified and digested sample DNA is loaded on a 0.8–1.0% agarose gel and the DNA fragments or topological forms are resolved by electrophoresis[87] (Figure 2.7). As DNA molecules are negatively charged, they migrate through the agarose matrix after an electric field is applied in a buffer chamber. The fixed pore size of the gel allows smaller fragments to move faster than larger ones. After electrophoresis, the agarose gel is first soaked in alkali to denature the DNA stands and then transferred by capillary blotting (the original Southern method) or by vacuum on to a nylon or nitrocellulose membrane. The DNA strands are then immobilized on the membrane by baking or by UV-mediated crosslinking, and the blot is hybridized to a labelled probe at the appropriate temperature. After washing, to remove non-specifically bound probe, the sample bands on a blot can be detected by autoradiography (radiolabel), fluorescent scan (fluorophore), chromogenic reaction or chemiluminescence (protein tags recognized by enzyme-conjugated antibodies). When HPV detection does not require concurrent HPV typing or the analysis of its replication status, purified sample DNA can be applied directly to a filter membrane. In such dot- or slot-blotting assays, the filter membrane is first treated and then the presence of HPV DNA visualized as described above for Southern blots.

In situ hybridization

This method permits the type-specific detection of HPV DNA directly in tissue sections from biopsies.[88] As with regular histological examinations, samples are first fixed, embed-

Figure 2.7
Southern blotting: this method and the related slot/dot blot assay are still widely used for detecting and typing HPVs. (a) Agarose gel electrophoresis: cellular/viral DNA mixtures are loaded in wells near the left edge. DNA molecules are negatively charged and will migrate to the right when an electric field is applied in a buffer chamber. The molecular sieving action of the agarose resolves the DNA fragments by size. Small fragments migrate faster towards the right edge of the gel. (b) Blotting: after denaturation of the DNAs the agarose gel is placed on a membrane filter that has affinity for DNA (nitrocellulose, nylon). Using capillary action or vacuum the single-stranded DNAs are transferred on to the membrane and immobilized (baking or UV irradiation). In slot/dot blotting, purified biopsy DNA is applied directly to the membrane filter and then also analysed as described in steps (c) and (d). (c) Hybridization: single-stranded DNA probes are labelled with nucleotides containing a radioactive (^{32}P, ^{35}S) or fluorescent (fluorescein, rhodamine) tag. During hybridization, the probe anneals to

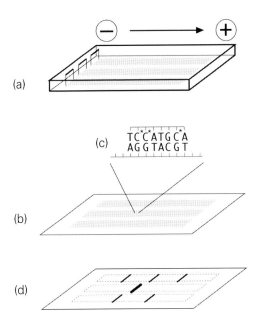

complementary sample sequences. Blots are then washed to remove non-specifically bound probe. (d) Detection: X-ray film (autoradiography for radioactive label) or a fluorescence imager (fluorescent label) is used to visualize the specific sample bands identified by the hybridized probe.

ded and sectioned. After removing the paraffin from the slides and making the tissue sections permeable, the resident sample DNAs are heat denatured and hybridized with labelled probes, similar to the description above for Southern blots.[87] Hybridized probes are usually detected chromogenically because it is more practical in the clinical laboratory setting than fluorescent or radioactive methods[90] (Figure 2.8).

Methods for the research laboratory

Many of the methods used in the clinical laboratory were originally developed for

research purposes and are still widely in use, such as PCR, Southern blotting and in situ hybridization. Typically, increased sensitivity and sophistication are gained by use of specialized laboratory equipment and more complex protocols.

Biochemistry

Generally, only the viral oncoproteins and capsid proteins are expressed at sufficiently high levels in HPV-infected tissue to permit direct detection by immunohistochemistry[81] or by immunoblot.[65] For this reason, biochemical studies aimed at determining the functions of

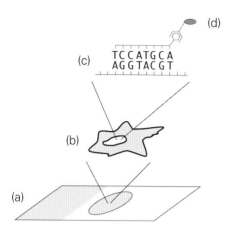

Figure 2.8

In situ hybridization: in contrast to the mass assays described above, in situ analysis identifies individual infected cells in the context of the biopsy tissue. It can also be used for HPV typing. (a) Sample slide: biopsy is fixed, sectioned and mounted. (b) Permeabilization: samples are treated with proteinase and detergent to provide probe access; the cellular DNA is heat denatured. (c) Hybridization: single-stranded DNA or RNA probes are labelled with nucleotides containing a radioactive (^{3}H, ^{35}S) or protein (biotin, digoxygenin) tag. During hybridization, the probe anneals to complementary sample sequences. Sample slides are then washed to remove non-specifically bound probe. (d) Detection: specific hybridization is visualized by (1) autoradiography (radioactive label) with a photoemulsion that is in direct contact with the sample; (2) chromogenic reaction of an enzyme that is conjugated to an antibody or avidin; or (3) fluorescence of a fluorophore-conjugated antibody or avidin.

the viral proteins use heterologous expression systems in bacteria, yeast, and mammalian or insect cells. Some of the viral regulatory proteins can be detected after metabolically

labelling HPV-infected cells and concentrating the labelled protein with a specific antibody in a radioimmunoprecipitation. Although the detection of viral proteins at their physiological levels is often not achievable, HPV-specific RNA and DNA can be analysed in all stages of viral infection with high sensitivity and accuracy. Southern blotting and PCR, as described above, are used for the detection of HPV DNA whereas viral RNA can be analysed by northern blotting, primer extension, RNase protection, or reverse-transcription (RT)-PCR. In situ hybridization, as described above, and in situ PCR are also used in the research laboratory for tissue-specific detection of viral DNA and RNA.

Cell culture

HPV biology can be studied in a variety of cell culture models. Cell culture-based research with recombinant HPV DNA has vastly increased our understanding of viral pathogenesis at the molecular level. The viral oncogenes of BPV1, the earliest prototype PV, were originally identified in transformation assays with murine fibroblasts which permitted a genetic analysis of the biology of the virus.[62,91] In contrast to BPV1, fibroblasts do not allow HPV replication[19] and, therefore, epithelial cells must be used for genetic studies. The immortalization capacity of high-risk HPV genomes for primary human keratinocytes[92] has allowed us to perform extensive analysis of their life cycle.[61,93,94] These methods can also be applied to study the biology of low-risk mucosal HPVs, taking into account that the resulting non-immortalized cells will eventually reach senescence.[95] With the exception of EV-specific HPVs[96,97] the biology of cutaneous types has not been studied extensively in cultured epithelial cells.[98]

One of the most valuable tools in HPV research is organotypic cell culture. High-risk

HPV-immortalized keratinocytes can be placed into this 'raft' system and allowed to form a stratified epithelium.[93] As a result of the faithful recapitulation of epithelial cell differentiation, which is a prerequisite for the productive stage of the HPV life cycle, genetic research with this model system has produced extensive insights into all phases of the viral life cycle.[12]

Animal models

The function of the HPV oncogenes can also be analysed in animal models. Although fibroblasts transformed with HPV oncogenes are tumorigenic in the nude mouse, HPV-immortalized keratinocytes require additional changes, which are induced by prolonged subculturing in vitro, before they acquire oncogenicity in this model. These findings support the notion that other cellular changes in addition to HPV oncogene expression are required for tumorigenicity.[99] Transgenic mice have also been used to analyse oncogene function in HPVs. Tissue-specific expression of high-risk E6 and E7 alters the normal developmental process of the target tissue and may also lead to the formation of tumours.[100,101] Such transgenic animal models are also useful for the study of the HPV-elicited immune response.[102,103]

Virus production

At present, there are no practical cell culture or animal systems that permit the generation of large numbers of HPV virions. Small numbers can be generated using the raft culture system.[104] HPV16 pseudotyped BPV1 virions have also been produced with a heterologous packaging system involving the Semliki-Forest virus-mediated expression of HPV capsid proteins.[105]

OUTLOOK

Papillomaviruses cause numerous benign and malignant human diseases. Although the analysis of their biology and pathogenesis initially lagged behind that of other viruses, because of the lack of a practical system for producing infectious virus for research, the methods of modern molecular biology largely overcame that limitation. To date, even the study of HPV-related immunology has gained sufficient momentum such that both the benign and the malignant consequences of HPV infection may soon be prevented or treated with vaccines.[106]

REFERENCES

1. zur Hausen H, de Villiers EM. Human papillomaviruses. *Annu Rev Microbiol* 1994; **48**: 427–47.
2. zur Hausen H. Papillomavirus infections – a major cause of human cancers. *Biochim Biophys Acta* 1996; **1288**: F55–78.
3. Howley PM. Papillomavirinae: The viruses and their replication. In: Fields BN, Knipe DM, Howley PM, eds. *Fundamental Virology*. Philadelphia: Lippincott-Raven, 1996: 947–78.
4. Belnap DM, Olson NH, Cladel NM et al. Conserved features in papillomavirus and polyomavirus capsids. *J Mol Biol* 1996; **259**: 249–63.
5. Baker TS, Newcomb WW, Olson NH, Cowsert LM, Olson C, Brown JC. Structures of bovine and human papillomaviruses. Analysis by cryoelectron microscopy and three-dimensional image reconstruction. *Biophys J* 1991; **60**: 1445–56.
6. Dyson N, Buchkovitch KPW, Harlow E. Cellular proteins that are targetted by DNA tumor viruses for transformation. *Princess Takamatsu Symp* 1989; **20**: 191–8.
7. Munger K, Werness BA, Dyson N, Phelps WC, Harlow E, Howley PM. Complex formation of human papillomavirus E7 proteins

with the retinoblastoma tumor suppressor gene product. *EMBO J* 1989; **8**: 4099–105.

8. Werness BA, Levine AJ, Howley PM. Association of human papillomavirus types 16 and 18 E6 proteins with p53. *Science* 1990; **248**: 76–9.

9. Vousden KH. Human papillomavirus oncoproteins. *Semin Cancer Biol* 1990; **1**: 415–24.

10. Tyring SK. Human papillomavirus infections: epidemiology, pathogenesis, and host immune response. *J Am Acad Dermatol* 2000; **43**: S18–S26.

11. Goldsborough MD, DiSilvestre D, Temple GF, Lorincz AT. Nucleotide sequence of human papillomavirus type 31: a cervical neoplasia-associated virus. *Virology* 1989; **171**: 306–11.

12. Laimins LA. Regulation of transcription and replication by human papillomaviruses. In: McCance DJ, ed. *Human Tumor Viruses*. American Society for Microbiology, 1998: 201–23.

13. Kanaya T, Kyo S, Laimins LA. The 5′ region of the human papillomavirus type 31 upstream regulatory region acts as an enhancer which augments viral early expression through the action of YY1. *Virology* 1997; **237**: 159–69.

14. Kyo S, Tam A, Laimins LA. Transcriptional activity of human papillomavirus type 31b enhancer is regulated through synergistic interaction of AP1 with two novel cellular factors. *Virology* 1995; **211**: 184–97.

15. Pattison S, Skalnik DG, Roman A. CCAAT displacement protein, a regulator of differentiation-specific gene expression, binds a negative regulatory element within the 5′ end of the human papillomavirus type 6 long control region. *J Virol* 1997; **71**: 2013–22.

16. Hubert WG, Kanaya T, Laimins LA. DNA replication of human papillomavirus type 31 is modulated by elements of the upstream regulatory region that lie 5′ of the minimal origin. *J Virol* 1999; **73**: 1835–45.

17. Steger G, Corbach S. Dose-dependent regulation of the early promoter of human papillomavirus type 18 by the viral E2 protein. *J Virol* 1997; **71**: 50–8.

18. Frattini MG, Laimins LA. The role of the E1 and E2 proteins in the replication of human papillomavirus type 31b. *Virology* 1994; **204**: 799–804.

19. Ustav M, Stenlund A. Transient replication of BPV-1 requires two viral polypeptides encoded by the E1 and E2 open reading frames. *EMBO J* 1991; **10**: 449–57.

20. Mohr IJ, Clark R, Sun S, Androphy EJ, MacPherson P, Botchan MR. Targeting the E1 replication protein to the papillomavirus origin of replication by complex formation with the E2 transactivator. *Science* 1990; **250**: 1694–9.

21. Yang L, Mohr I, Fouts E, Lim DA, Nohaile M, Botchan M. The E1 protein of bovine papilloma virus 1 is an ATP-dependent DNA helicase. *Proc Natl Acad Sci USA* 1993; **90**: 5086–90.

22. Lambert PF, Hubbert NL, Howley PM, Schiller JT. Genetic assignment of multiple E2 gene products in bovine papillomavirus-transformed cells. *J Virol* 1989; **63**: 3151–4.

23. Stubenrauch F, Hummel M, Iftner T, Laimins LA. The E8E2C protein, a negative regulator of viral transcription and replication, is required for extrachromosomal maintenance of human papillomavirus type 31 in keratinocytes. *J Virol* 2000; **74**: 1178–86.

24. Dyson N, Guida P, Munger K, Harlow E. Homologous sequences in adenovirus E1A and human papillomavirus E7 proteins mediate interaction with the same set of cellular proteins. *J Virol* 1992; **66**: 6893–902.

25. Tommasino M, Adamczewski JP, Carlotti F et al. HPV16 E7 protein associates with the protein kinase p33CDK2 and cyclin A. *Oncogene* 1993; **8**: 195–202.

26. McIntyre MC, Ruesch MN, Laimins LA. Human papillomavirus E7 oncoproteins bind a single form of cyclin E in a complex with cdk2 and p107. *Virology* 1996; **215**: 73–82.

27. Jones DL, Alani RM, Munger K. The human papillomavirus E7 oncoprotein can uncouple

cellular differentiation and proliferation in human keratinocytes by abrogating p21Cip1–mediated inhibition of cdk2. *Genes Dev* 1997; **11**: 2101–11.

28. Funk JO, Waga S, Harry JB, Espling E, Stillman B, Galloway DA. Inhibition of CDK activity and PCNA-dependent DNA replication by p21 is blocked by interaction with the HPV-16 E7 oncoprotein. *Genes Dev* 1997; **11**: 2090–100.

29. Zerfass-Thome K, Zwerschke W, Mannhardt B, Tindle R, Botz JW, Jansen-Durr P. Inactivation of the cdk inhibitor p27KIP1 by the human papillomavirus type 16 E7 oncoprotein. *Oncogene* 1996; **13**: 2323–30.

30. Davies R, Hicks R, Crook T, Morris J, Vousden K. Human papillomavirus type 16 E7 associates with a histone H1 kinase and with p107 through sequences necessary for transformation. *J Virol* 1993; **67**: 25218.

31. Brehm A, Nielsen SJ, Miska EA et al. The E7 oncoprotein associates with Mi2 and histone deacetylase activity to promote cell growth. *EMBO J* 1999; **18**: 2449–58.

32. Antinore MJ, Birrer MJ, Patel D, Nader L, McCance DJ. The human papillomavirus type 16 E7 gene product interacts with and transactivates the AP1 family of transcription factors. *EMBO J* 1996; **15**: 1950–60.

33. Gage JR, Meyers C, Wettstein FO. The E7 proteins of the nononcogenic human papillomavirus type 6b (HPV- 6b) and of the oncogenic HPV-16 differ in retinoblastoma protein binding and other properties. *J Virol* 1990; **64**: 723–30.

34. Zehbe I, Ratsch A et al. Overriding of cyclin-dependent kinase inhibitors by high and low risk human papillomavirus types: evidence for an in vivo role in cervical lesions. *Oncogene* 1999; **18**: 2201–11.

35. Rapp L, Chen JJ. The papillomavirus E6 proteins. *Biochim Biophys Acta* 1998; **1378**: F1–F19.

36. Huibregtse JM, Scheffner M, Howley PM. A cellular protein mediates association of p53 with the E6 oncoprotein of human papillomavirus types 16 or 18. *EMBO J* 1991; **10**: 4129–35.

37. Kukimoto I, Aihara S, Yoshiike K, Kanda T. Human papillomavirus oncoprotein E6 binds to the C-terminal region of human minichromosome maintenance 7 protein. *Biochem Biophys Res Commun* 1998; **249**: 258–62.

38. Kuhne C, Banks L. E3–ubiquitin ligase/E6-AP links multicopy maintenance protein 7 to the ubiquitination pathway by a novel motif, the L2G box. *J Biol Chem* 1998; **273**: 34302–9.

39. Patel D, Huang SM, Baglia LA, McCance DJ. The E6 protein of human papillomavirus type 16 binds to and inhibits co-activation by CBP and p300. *EMBO J* 1999; **18**: 5061–72.

40. Zimmermann H, Degenkolbe R, Bernard HU, O'Connor MJ. The human papillomavirus type 16 E6 oncoprotein can down-regulate p53 activity by targeting the transcriptional coactivator CBP/p300. *J Virol* 1999; **73**: 6209–19.

41. Kiyono T, Hiraiwa A, Fujita M, Hayashi Y, Akiyama T, Ishibashi M. Binding of high-risk human papillomavirus E6 oncoproteins to the human homologue of the Drosophila discs large tumor suppressor protein. *Proc Natl Acad Sci USA* 1997; **94**: 11612–16.

42. Lee SS, Weiss RS, Javier RT. Binding of human virus oncoproteins to hDlg/SAP97, a mammalian homolog of the Drosophila discs large tumor suppressor protein. *Proc Natl Acad Sci USA* 1997; **94**: 6670–5.

43. Gao Q, Srinivasan S, Boyer SN, Wazer DE, Band V. The E6 oncoproteins of high-risk papillomaviruses bind to a novel putative GAP protein, E6TP1, and target it for degradation. *Mol Cell Biol* 1999; **19**: 733–44.

44. Chen JJ, Reid CE, Band V, Androphy EJ. Interaction of papillomavirus E6 oncoproteins with a putative calcium-binding protein. *Science* 1995; **269**: 529–31.

45. Tong X, Howley PM. The bovine papillomavirus E6 oncoprotein interacts with paxillin and disrupts the actin cytoskeleton. *Proc Natl Acad Sci USA* 1997; **94**: 4412–17.

46. Tong X, Boll W, Kirchhausen T, Howley PM. Interaction of the bovine papillomavirus E6

protein with the clathrin adaptor complex AP-1. *J Virol* 1998; **72**: 476–82.

47. Ronco LV, Karpova AY, Vidal M, Howley PM. Human papillomavirus 16 E6 oncoprotein binds to interferon regulatory factor-3 and inhibits its transcriptional activity. *Genes Dev* 1998; **12**: 2061–72.

48. Li S, Labrecque S, Gauzzi MC et al. The human papilloma virus (HPV)-18 E6 oncoprotein physically associates with Tyk2 and impairs Jak-STAT activation by interferon-alpha. *Oncogene* 1999; **18**: 5727–37.

49. Goldstein DJ, Finbow ME, Andresson T, McLean P, Smith K, Bubb V et al. Bovine papillomavirus E5 oncoprotein binds to the 16K component of vacuolar H(+)-ATPases. *Nature* 1991; **352**: 347–9.

50. Conrad M, Bubb VJ, Schlegel R. The human papillomavirus type 6 and 16 E5 proteins are membrane-associated proteins which associate with the 16-kilodalton pore-forming protein. *J Virol* 1993; **67**: 6170–8.

51. Straight SW, Hinkle PM, Jewers RJ, McCance DJ. The E5 oncoprotein of human papillomavirus type 16 transforms fibroblasts and effects the downregulation of the epidermal growth factor receptor in keratinocytes. *J Virol* 1993; **67**: 4521–32.

52. Farmer A, Myers G. E5 nucleotide and protein alignment. In: Myers G, ed. *Human Papillomavirus 1997 Compendium*. Los Alamos, NM: Los Alamos National Laboratory, 1997: II-E5-1.

53. Doorbar J, Campbell D, Grand RJ, Gallimore PH. Identification of the human papilloma virus-1a E4 gene products. *EMBO J* 1986; **5**: 355–62.

54. Doorbar J, Ely S, Sterling J, McLean C, Crawford L. Specific interaction between HPV-16 E1–E4 and cytokeratins results in collapse of the epithelial cell intermediate filament network. *Nature* 1991; **352**: 824–7.

55. Kirnbauer R, Taub J, Greenstone H et al. Efficient self-assembly of human papillomavirus type 16 L1 and L1–L2 into virus-like particles. *J Virol* 1993; **67**: 6929–36.

56. Day PM, Roden RB, Lowy DR, Schiller JT. The papillomavirus minor capsid protein, L2, induces localization of the major capsid protein, L1, and the viral transcription/replication protein, E2, to PML oncogenic domains. *J Virol* 1998; **72**: 142–50.

57. Kawana Y, Kawana K, Yoshikawa H, Taketani Y, Yoshiike K, Kanda T. Human papillomavirus type 16 minor capsid protein l2 N-terminal region containing a common neutralization epitope binds to the cell surface and enters the cytoplasm. *J Virol* 2001; **75**: 2331–6.

58. Evander M, Frazer IH, Payne E, Qi YM, Hengst K, McMillan NA. Identification of the alpha6 integrin as a candidate receptor for papillomaviruses. *J Virol* 1997; **71**: 2449–56.

59. McMillan NA, Payne E, Frazer IH, Evander M. Expression of the alpha6 integrin confers papillomavirus binding upon receptor-negative B-cells. *Virology* 1999; **261**: 271–9.

60. Giroglou T, Florin L, Schafer F, Streeck RE, Sapp M. Human papillomavirus infection requires cell surface heparan sulfate. *J Virol* 2001; **75**: 1565–70.

61. Frattini MG, Lim HB, Laimins LA. In vitro synthesis of oncogenic human papillomaviruses requires episomal genomes for differentiation-dependent late expression. *Proc Natl Acad Sci USA* 1996; **93**: 3062–7.

62. Dvoretzky I, Shober R, Chattopadhyay SK, Lowy DR. A quantitative in vitro focus assay for bovine papilloma virus. *Virology* 1980; **103**: 369–75.

63. Gilbert DM, Cohen SN. Bovine papilloma virus plasmids replicate randomly in mouse fibroblasts throughout S phase of the cell cycle. *Cell* 1987; **50**: 59–68.

64. Romanczuk H, Howley PM. Disruption of either the E1 or the E2 regulatory gene of human papillomavirus type 16 increases viral immortalization capacity. *Proc Natl Acad Sci USA* 1992; **89**: 3159–63.

65. Jeon S, Allen-Hoffmann BL, Lambert PF. Integration of human papillomavirus type 16 into the human genome correlates with a

selective growth advantage of cells. *J Virol* 1995; **69**: 2989–97.

66. Durst M, Kleinheinz A, Hotz M, Gissman L. The physical state of human papillomavirus type 16 DNA in benign and malignant genital tumours. *J Gen Virol* 1985; **66**: 1515–22.

67. Jeon S, Lambert PF. Integration of human papillomavirus type 16 DNA into the human genome leads to increased stability of E6 and E7 mRNAs: implications for cervical carcinogenesis. *Proc Natl Acad Sci USA* 1995; **92**: 1654–8.

68. Vilcek J, Sen GC. Interferons and other cytokines. In: Fields BN, Knipe DM, Howley PM, eds, *Fields Virology*, 3rd edn. Philadelphia: Lippincott-Raven, 1996: 375–99.

69. Darnell JE Jr, Kerr IM, Stark GR. Jak-STAT pathways and transcriptional activation in response to IFNs and other extracellular signaling proteins. *Science* 1994; **264**: 1415–21.

70. Stark GR, Kerr IM. Interferon-dependent signaling pathways: DNA elements, transcription factors, mutations, and effects of viral proteins. *J Interferon Res* 1992; **12**: 147–51.

71. Bluyssen AR, Durbin JE, Levy DE. ISGF3 gamma p48, a specificity switch for interferon activated transcription factors. *Cytokine Growth Factor Rev* 1996; **7**: 11–17.

72. Barnard P, McMillan NA. The human papillomavirus E7 oncoprotein abrogates signaling mediated by interferon-alpha. *Virology* 1999; **259**: 305–13.

73. Frazer IH, Thomas R, Zhou J et al. Potential strategies utilised by papillomavirus to evade host immunity. *Immunol Rev* 1999; **168**: 131–42.

74. Shah KV, Howley PM. Papillomaviruses. In: Fields BN, Knipe DM, Howley PM, eds, *Fields Virology*, 3rd edn. Philadelphia: Lippincott-Raven, 1996: 2077–109.

75. Da Silva DM, Eiben GL, Fausch SC et al. Cervical cancer vaccines: emerging concepts and developments. *J Cell Physiol* 2001; **186**: 169–82.

76. Zeller R. Fixation, embedding, and sectioning of tissues, embryos, and single cells. In: Ausubel FM, Brent R, Kingston RE et al, eds, *Current Protocols in Molecular Biology*. New York: John Wiley & Sons, 1989: 14.1.1–8.

77. Watkins S. Cryosectioning. In: Ausubel FM, Brent R, Kingston RE et al, eds, *Current Protocols in Molecular Biology*. New York: John Wiley & Sons, 1989: 14.2.1–8.

78. Mitchell MF, Tortolero-Luna G, Wright T et al. Cervical human papillomavirus infection and intraepithelial neoplasia: a review. *J Natl Cancer Inst Monogr* 1996; **21**: 17–25.

79. Perlman SE. Pap smears: screening, interpretation, treatment. *Adolesc Med* 1999; **10**: 243–54.

80. Digene Corporation. HC2(r) Hybrid Capture System for HPV detection. http://www.digene.com/lifesciences_2_1_1.html (March 2002).

81. Meyers C, Frattini MG, Hudson JB, Laimins LA. Biosynthesis of human papillomavirus from a continuous cell line upon epithelial differentiation. *Science* 1992; **257**: 971–3.

82. Kramer MF, Coen DM. Enzymatic amplification of DNA by PCR: Standard procedures and optimization. In: Ausubel FM, Brent R, Kingston RE et al, eds, *Current Protocols in Molecular Biology*. New York: John Wiley & Sons, 1999: 15.1.1–14.

83. Shamanin V, Delius H, de Villiers EM. Development of a broad spectrum PCR assay for papillomaviruses and its application in screening lung cancer biopsies. *J Gen Virol* 1994; **75**: 1149–56.

84. Shamanin V, zur Hausen H, Lavergne D et al. Human papillomavirus infections in nonmelanoma skin cancers from renal transplant recipients and nonimmunosuppressed patients. *J Natl Cancer Inst* 1996; **88**: 802–11.

85. de Villiers EM, Lavergne D, McLaren K, Benton EC. Prevailing papillomavirus types in non-melanoma carcinomas of the skin in renal allograft recipients. *Int J Cancer* 1997; **73**: 356–61.

86. Harwood CA, Spink PJ, Surentheran T et al. Degenerate and nested PCR: a highly sensitive and specific method for detection of human papillomavirus infection in cutaneous warts. *J Clin Microbiol* 1999; **37**: 3545–55.

87. Brown T. Southern blotting. In: Ausubel FM, Brent R, Kingston RE et al, eds, *Current Protocols in Molecular Biology*. New York: John Wiley & Sons, 1993: 2.9.1–15.

88. Zeller R. In situ hybridization to cellular RNA. In: Ausubel FM, Brent R, Kingston RE et al, eds, *Current Protocols in Molecular Biology*. New York: John Wiley & Sons, 1989: 14.3.1–14.

89. Rogers M. Detection of hybridized probe. In: Ausubel FM, Brent R, Kingston RE et al, eds, *Current Protocols in Molecular Biology*. New York: John Wiley & Sons, 1989: 14.4.1–3.

90. Knoll JHM. In situ hybridization and detection using nonisotopic probes. In: Ausubel FM, Brent R, Kingston RE et al, eds, *Current Protocols in Molecular Biology*. New York: John Wiley & Sons, 1995: 14.7.1–14.

91. Lambert PF. Papillomavirus DNA replication. *J Virol* 1991; **65**: 3417–20.

92. Munger K, Phelps WC, Bubb V, Howley PM, Schlegel R. The E6 and E7 genes of the human papillomavirus type 16 together are necessary and sufficient for transformation of primary human keratinocytes. *J Virol* 1989; **63**: 4417–21.

93. Meyers C, Laimins LA. In vitro systems for the study and propagation of human papillomaviruses. *Curr Top Microbiol Immunol* 1994; **186**: 199–215.

94. Frattini MG, Lim HB, Doorbar J, Laimins LA. Induction of human papillomavirus type 18 late gene expression and genomic amplification in organotypic cultures from transfected DNA templates. *J Virol* 1997; **71**: 7068–72.

95. Thomas JT, Oh ST, Terhune SS, Laimins LA. Cellular changes induced by low-risk human papillomavirus type 11 in keratinocytes that stably maintain viral episomes. *J Virol* 2001; **75**: 7564–71.

96. Reh H, Pfister H. Human papillomavirus type 8 contains cis-active positive and negative transcriptional control sequences. *J Gen Virol* 1990; **71**: 2457–62.

97. Enzenauer C, Mengus G, Lavigne A, Davidson I, Pfister H, May M. Interaction of human papillomavirus 8 regulatory proteins E2, E6 and E7 with components of the TFIID complex. *Intervirology* 1998; **41**: 80–90.

98. Williams AT, Sexton CJ, Sinclair AL et al. Retention of low copy number human papillomavirus DNA in cultured cutaneous and mucosal wart keratinocytes. *J Gen Virol* 1994; **75**: 505–11.

99. Durst M, Seagon S, Wanschura S, zur Hausen H, Bullerdiek J. Malignant progression of an HPV16-immortalized human keratinocyte cell line (HPKIA) in vitro. *Cancer Genet Cytogenet* 1995; **85**: 105–12.

100. Griep AE, Herber R, Jeon S, Lohse JK, Dubielzig RR, Lambert PF. Tumorigenicity by human papillomavirus type 16 E6 and E7 in transgenic mice correlates with alterations in epithelial cell growth and differentiation. *J Virol* 1993; **67**: 1373–84.

101. Lambert PF, Pan H, Pitot HC, Liem A, Jackson M, Griep AE. Epidermal cancer associated with expression of human papillomavirus type 16 E6 and E7 oncogenes in the skin of transgenic mice. *Proc Natl Acad Sci USA* 1993; **90**: 5583–7.

102. Frazer IH, Leippe DM, Dunn LA et al. Immunological responses in human papillomavirus 16 E6/E7-transgenic mice to E7 protein correlate with the presence of skin disease. *Cancer Res* 1995; **55**: 2635–9.

103. Hilditch-Maguire PA, Lieppe DM, West D, Lambert PF, Frazer IH. T cell-mediated and non-specific inflammatory mechanisms contribute to the skin pathology of HPV 16 E6E7 transgenic mice. *Intervirology* 1999; **42**: 43–50.

104. Meyers C, Mayer TJ, Ozbun MA. Synthesis of infectious human papillomavirus type 18 in differentiating epithelium transfected with viral DNA. *J Virol* 1997; **71**: 7381–6.

105. Roden RB, Greenstone HL, Kirnbauer R et al. In vitro generation and type-specific neutralization of a human papillomavirus type 16 virion pseudotype. *J Virol* 1996; **70**: 5875–83.

106. zur Hausen H. Cervical carcinoma and human papillomavirus: on the road to preventing a major human cancer. *J Natl Cancer Inst* 2001; **93**: 252–3.

3 Epidemiology

E Brian Russell

Historical aspects • Background • Cutaneous HPV infections in the normal host • Infection in the immunocompromised host • Mucosal and sexually transmitted HPV infections • Conclusion • References

The human papillomavirus (HPV) has a wide range of clinical manifestations, from benign cutaneous nuisances to life-threatening cellular transformations. As the science in this area progresses, we are often left with more questions than answers. Nowhere is this more true than in the area of HPV epidemiology. Currently, there are at least 83 unique types of HPV characterized by DNA sequencing.[1] In addition, over 150 types have been identified by the polymerase chain reaction (PCR). As these viruses are split into finer and finer genotypic categories, we find that there is often considerable overlap in their phenotypic characteristics yielding clinically indistinguishable infections, e.g. at least 15 types of HPV are associated with cervical carcinoma.[2] This chapter is devoted to: (1) placing HPV epidemiology into historical perspective; (2) providing background information on the way epidemiological data are gathered; (3) analysing current trends in cutaneous HPV infections both in the normal host and in the immunocompromised patient; and (4) presenting the current data about mucosal and sexually transmitted HPV infections.

HISTORICAL ASPECTS

Most sexually transmitted diseases (STDs) have a relatively short history, e.g. the Italian poet Fracastoro described syphilis, one of the older venereal diseases, in the sixteenth century.[3] HPV in the form of condyloma acuminata may be traced much further back in time – to at least 2000 years ago.[4] Roman cultures were very familiar with this disease, and philosophers made reference to both common warts and condyloma. Martial in the first century even speculated on the communicable nature of the latter (Figure 3.1).[5]

In spite of recognizing that warts were contagious, it was not until the last century that the nature of the offending agent was defined. Wile and Kingery[6] sought to disprove the dogma in 1919 that verrucae were caused by a bacterial agent. Earlier experiments by Jadassohn in 1894, in which he inoculated keratinocytes from warts into healthy volunteer skin and produced verrucae, were cited as pivotal in establishing an infectious aetiology. However, Wile and Kingery were able to lyse keratinocytes, filter the lysates, and successfully re-infect themselves and their assistants

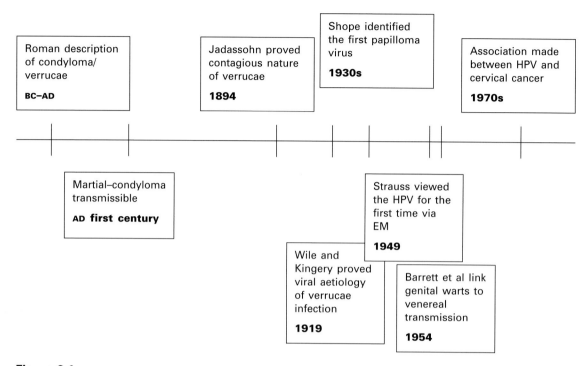

Figure 3.1
An HPV historical timeline.

with the ultrafiltrates. They concluded that common warts were caused by a virus.[6] Papillomavirus was identified as a cotton-tail rabbit pathogen in the 1930s.[7] The cotton-tail rabbit papillomavirus produced tumors in their hosts, and this was the first DNA virus to demonstrate transformation properties in a mammalian system. An advance in technology, electron microscopy, altered and furthered the burgeoning field of virology in the middle of the twentieth century. This device enabled Strauss to view the viral elements of HPV in 1949.[8]

A few years later, another important study focused on the venereal transmission of genital warts.[9] This subject had been discussed in the literature years before this conclusive treatise. These military physicians observed soldiers returning from Korea: 70 soldiers with no history of condylomata before their tours developed clinical infections; 94% admitted to having intercourse while in the Far East. A large portion (at least one-third) of these patients reported that their wives subsequently developed genital warts, adding finality to the notion of sexual transmission.

BACKGROUND

As alluded to earlier, the large numbers of different papillomaviruses lead to protean clinical manifestations. There are a number of

Table 3.1 Phenotypic expressions and human papillomavirus type

Risk	HPV type
High	16, 18
Moderate	31, 33, 35, 39, 45, 51, 52, 53, 55, 56, 58, 59, 63, 66, 68
Low	6, 11, 42, 43, 44

categories of infection, all of which stem from the virus's predilection for squamous epithelium. As far as we know, successful HPV infection is limited to the keratinocyte.[10] HPV disease may be most effectively categorized based on involvement of cornified versus mucosal surfaces (there are overlaps within these categories). Within each of these divisions, there is a wide range of clinical findings from common verrucous papules on the finger of a child to aggressive epithelioma cuniculatum, or from the focal epithelial hyperplasia of Heck to invasive genital squamous cell carcinoma. Table 3.1 features the different phenotypic expressions along with their associated HPV types. It is notable that some HPVs have limited potential for infecting the different epithelial surfaces in the human host, whereas others such as HPV6 and -11 are found in cornified or mucosal epithelium.[2,11] This diversity among the HPVs creates great difficulty in epidemiological study, although other variables are perhaps even more confounding. First among these is the high rate of subclinical and undetectable infections.[8,10,12] This is analysed later in greater detail. Another barrier is the inadequacy of current laboratory methods for viral study. The virus has over 20 different hosts, but it is species specific and there is no animal model for human infection.[13] Not only is there no model, there is also no way to grow the particles in culture. The virus requires differentiated keratinocytes for successful inoculation, but, in

a classic catch 22 circumstance, differentiated keratinocytes do not replicate.[10] A number of techniques are emerging to circumvent these issues, and these are discussed more thoroughly in Chapter 2. Finally, the disease is not classified as reportable to health agencies, so data from broad populations are not readily obtained.[1]

There are many ways to classify an HPV infection. First and foremost is the clinical examination. A number of studies on the prevalence of cutaneous verrucae have been performed on this basis alone.[14] Histopathology often adds significantly to the diagnostic accuracy of the clinician, and the advent of the Papanicolaou smear and the customary use of biopsies in suspicious lesions have greatly reduced the mortality rates of cervical cancer in the USA.[15]

Serological studies are most often performed in large population surveys. These studies usually seek to determine the prevalence of HPV in their participants.[16–18] The method is valuable in detecting remote infections in people who may have cleared the virus, because antibodies remain indefinitely. However, one drawback of such studies is that all those who have detectable antibodies are counted as HPV exposed, no matter the extent (or lack thereof) of clinical infection. Another disadvantage to consider is the specificity of the antibody detection systems. Hosts develop antibodies primarily to the capsid proteins of HPV, and these are virus specific. Therefore individual HPV capsid proteins against which human antibodies develop must be manufactured, mass produced and commercially available for serological studies. Obviously, this is possible only with a small number of HPVs. Of note, both cell-mediated immunity and humoral immunity may be required to clear HPV. By measuring antibodies to HPV, one may not capture all those who have been infected with HPV.

In the past, studies have used electron microscopy for gathering epidemiological data.[19,20] However, the technique is now rarely used for this purpose, because more sensitive and less technically demanding procedures are now available.[21,22]

Molecular biology has provided new and more complex means of HPV identification. DNA hybridization and PCR are the newest and most sensitive methods. Most studies using these procedures focus on identifying new viruses or on recognizing viral subtypes in diseased tissue. Nucleic acid hybridization assays are sensitive and specific for HPV. Southern blot hybridization is the most accurate of these methods; however, it is also the most demanding of the hybridization techniques and not suited to widespread

epidemiological application.[7] The technique of *in situ* hybridization sacrifices some of the precision of the Southern blot, but enables direct visualization of infected cells.[7] This is a tool that is most frequently employed in tissue-limited situations and experiments determining the presence of virus in affected versus adjoining unaffected skin.[7]

The PCR has significantly advanced the study of papillomaviruses. It is the most sensitive method for viral identification, and there are myriad applications for this tool, including identification of new agents, typing of viral particles in diseased tissue to determine prognosis and treatment, and broad-reaching prevalence studies[8] (Figure 3.2). A number of reports cited later in this chapter make use of PCR for generation of epidemiological data, and one such application is shown in Figure 3.2. A more detailed analysis of these techniques and their application to the study of HPV may be found in Chapter 2.

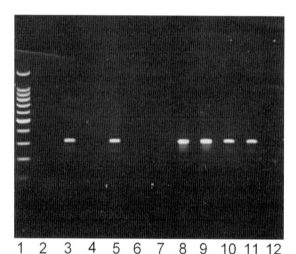

Figure 3.2
An example of the use of the polymerase chain reaction for the identification of human papillomavirus (HPV). In these cases, lane 1 represents a ladder control and lane 12 a negative control. The experimental groups in lanes 2–11 represent tissue from patients in our centre who had verrucae vulgaris clinically. The bands in lanes 3, 5 and 8–11 are positive for HPV group A4, which consists of viral types 2, 27 and 57.

CUTANEOUS HPV INFECTIONS IN THE NORMAL HOST

Cutaneous manifestations in epidemiological terms in the immunocompetent individual are very different from those in the immunologically compromised host, so these topics are discussed separately. The number of papers devoted to the study of cutaneous HPV pales in comparison with STDs. However, there have been a number of quality studies performed, primarily aimed at documenting the prevalence of common, plantar and plane verrucae in communities. In addition, there have been new links established between HPV and previously idiopathic skin findings, e.g. HPV6 and -11 were found in 88% of fibroepithelial polyps by Dianzani et al.[11] Data have also been gathered with specific high-risk groups such as poultry workers and users of communal showers, which show them to be more likely to develop butcher's warts and verrucae plantaris, respectively.[23,24] A meta-analysis of the literature relating to wart prevalence in communities revealed that infection rates varied depending on the population considered.[14] The rates in children were between 2% and 20%. These numbers are mirrored in more recent studies. In Romania, 1114 school children aged 6–12 had a point prevalence of non-genital viral verrucae of 2.8%.[25] In an Australian study by the above author (Kilkenny), 2491 children demonstrated a much higher rate of warts.[26] In the 4- to 12-year age range the prevalence was between 12.5% and 25%. The older children aged between 10 and 18 years had higher rates than the younger children. Other important conclusions from the meta-analysis included a lack of sex variation for warts (except perhaps in verrucae plantaris, which showed the female sex to be more at risk) and predominance in white versus black individuals.

Reports on the natural history of HPV are more comprehensive with mucosal disease (see 'HPV infection of the anogenital region'). The classic information from a 2-year prospective study of patients with cutaneous verrucae showed that involution of individual warts occurs in two-thirds of the cases over this time period, although those having warts were at higher risk for developing new ones.[27] At the end of the 2 years, 46% of the patients with verrucae were free of disease. None of the study participants developed more significant or harmful manifestations. However, findings of tumorigenic HPVs in extragenital squamous cell carcinoma are becoming more frequent.[28–30] None of these studies identified a precursor verrucous papule before the development of the malignancy, so it must be concluded that these HPV-related cancers developed from new infections. Further exploration of HPV's role in cutaneous malignancy is presented in the next section.

INFECTION IN THE IMMUNOCOMPROMISED HOST

The immune status of a patient is always important when considering a communicable disease such as HPV. As with most other infections, HPV is more severe and debilitating when the immune system is suppressed.

Certainly there are a number of conditions that predispose a patient to HPV infection, and perhaps the most prominently represented in the dermatology clinic is the solid organ transplant recipient. Chronic anti-rejection measures with corticosteroids, azathioprine, cyclosporin, etc. leave cell-mediated immunity deficient. This enables a ubiquitous virus such as HPV to establish unusually high rates of infection. In a British analysis of 291 renal transplant recipients, an overall prevalence of cutaneous verrucae was established at 59%.[30a] However, perhaps even more impressive was the 90% rate obtained for patients more than 5 years after their transplantation. The clinical manifestations tend to be more extensive in this population and the viral subtypes are often different from the classic descriptions.[31]

The development of skin cancers in transplant recipients is quite common. Researchers have tried with disparate results to link this finding to the presence of HPV.[31–33] More recently, Harwood et al[34] used a PCR technique with broad applicability to the various HPV types and demonstrated HPV in a large portion of the immuno-suppressed patients' non-melanoma skin cancers. Interestingly, a disproportionately high number of these HPV types were 5 and 8 – the types most associated with another immuno-suppressed state, epidermodysplasia verruciformis. Thus, it seems likely that papillomavirus plays a part in the aetiology of skin cancer in the iatrogenic immunocompromised patient.

The patient infected with the human immunodeficiency virus (HIV) is similar to the transplant recipient – both have inadequate cell-mediated immune surveillance, with the consequence that the rates of cutaneous HPV infection are similar between these groups. The rates for anogenital carcinomas are much higher, however, in the HIV population, which is not surprising given the sexual transmission characteristics of both agents.[35] In addition, cervical cancer in HIV-positive women is now listed as an acquired immune deficiency syndrome (AIDS)-defining condition.[35] This is almost certainly HPV related. Not only are prevalences for warts higher than in the normal population, but the types of HPVs involved are also unusual.[36] Patients with HIV also develop more oral and gastrointestinal HPV infections than immunocompetent individuals.[37]

Epidermodysplasia verruciformis is a rare inherited condition recently mapped in families to chromosomes 2 and 17.[38,39] Individuals with this autosomal recessive genodermatosis have been found to have specific deficits in cell-mediated immunity, while having increased peripheral natural killer cell activity and normal humoral defences.[40] The deficient T-cell immunity predisposes EV patients to subtypes of HPV infection, namely HPV5 and -8. However, at least 21 others have been described.[13] Clinical manifestations of this disease are fairly narrow when compared with other immunocompromised states. Keratotic papules on the dorsa of the hands and scaling, erythematous macules on the trunk are the hallmarks, with slow evolution of the lesions towards Bowen's disease and eventually foci of squamous cell carcinoma.[41] Sunlight, which depresses local immunity and damages DNA, appears to induce cancer in these predisposed patients. The malignancies do not have a propensity to metastasize unless irradiated (similar to verrucous carcinoma).[13]

MUCOSAL AND SEXUALLY TRANSMITTED HPV INFECTIONS

The distinction between mucosal disease and an STD is often a difficult one to make. Sexual habits over the years have changed, blurring the once clear division between non-sexually acquired, predominantly head and neck diseases and venereal diseases. The classic example is seen with herpes virus infections. In years past, herpes simplex type 1 was equated with herpes labialis and type 2 was responsible for genital disease. Although this is still the case in most situations, this transmission should not be presumed.[42] Such is the case with HPV. With that point in mind, this section is divided for the sake of simplicity between infections of the head and neck mucosae and infections of the anogenital regions.

HPV infection of the head and neck

The link between HPV and oral malignancy has not been firmly established. Most tumors of the aerodigestive tracts have been primarily associated with physical and chemical insults such as tobacco and ethanol. However, studies are emerging that reveal multifactorial associations, including identification of numerous HPV types, with oropharyngeal carcinomas as well as with benign, polypoid tumors.[43–45] These findings are tempered by other reports that demonstrate viral elements in clinically normal hosts.[46–48] A variant of verrucous carcinoma, oral florid papillomatosis, is comparable histologically to the genital Buschke–Lowenstein tumor caused by HPV6/11. Although the papillomavirus is thought to be involved in this oral carcinoma, this fact has yet to be proved.[13]

Archard, Heck and Stanley first described a rare familial syndrome now known as Heck's disease in 1965. This disorder has been shown primarily in Native Americans and presents clinically as small, 1–5 mm, flesh-colored papules on the lips, gingivae and buccal mucosae.[13] HPV13 has been uniquely demonstrated in Heck's papillomas, but HPV1, -18 and -32 have also been found in the lesions.[1,49] There is no known transformation of the disease to malignancy.

Finally, ocular papillomas have also been shown to contain HPV. McDonnell et al[50] studied 23 conjunctival papillomas using DNA hybridization techniques and found that 65% were positive for type 6. However, the viral particles were limited to benign neoplasms as none of the 28 histologically dysplastic lesions demonstrated HPV.

HPV infection of the anogenital region

The Centers for Disease Control and Prevention state that 'HPV is likely the most common STD among young, sexually active people'.[51] Their data currently assume an annual infection rate in the USA of 5.5 million. Currently, there are at least 20 million individuals estimated to have transmissible infections. Cates[52] estimated that, in 1996, HPV and another frequent infection of the genital tract, trichomoniasis, accounted for more than two-thirds of STDs in the USA. Although genital HPV is usually thought of as a disease of women, it has been documented that infection rates between the sexes are similar.[53] In this section, the illnesses of men and women are discussed separately, because the morbidity and mortality differ. The distinctions among viral exposure, subclinical infection and frank clinical disease are also emphasized.

Important points to consider when studying the epidemiology of a communicable agent are infectivity and transmissibility. The number of infective virions in the cutaneous wart is much greater than in genital warts. However, the transmission of HPV via mucosal contact is very efficient, and the virus maintains its capacity for infection in spite of desiccation.[42,54,55] As a result, there are findings of fomite and hand–genital spread of HPV.[56–58]

Fortunately, the successful clearance rate for mucosal infection is around 70% a year after exposure.[55] As mentioned earlier, the epidemiology of HPV may focus on exposure to the virus (usually measured with serological assays) or on active or subclinical infections (usually determined with tissue sampling).

The important link in humans between HPV and cervical cancer began about 25 years ago and has since become an area of intense research.[10,59] Invasive cervical malignancies are 90–95% likely to contain identifiable HPV DNA.[35] Significant advances have been achieved by women's health providers in developed countries in the area of early detection of potentially life-threatening invasive disease; however, cervical cancer remains the second most common cause of malignancy-related death among women in the world.[10,60] In general, the HPV types associated with genital tract carcinoma are divided into several categories, with HPV16 accounting for 50% of the total (Table 3.1).[2,61] The link between sexually acquired HPV and genital carcinoma is strong. Studies of women who are sexually active show high rates of HPV infections and, with greater numbers of partners, the higher the risk.[16,62–64] Barrier devices that prevent mucosal contact and fluid exchange decrease infection rates, whereas chemical and oral contraceptives may be associated with higher rates of infection.[65,66] In addition, virgins are at negligible, if any, risk for HPV and cervical cancer.[18,67]

Although HPV infection is the most important risk factor for developing cervical carcinoma, it is clear that it is not the only one. The natural history of infection, especially subclinical disease, is overwhelmingly in favour of complete resolution.[63] In their study, Ho et al[63] observed women over a 3-year span. They found that, after acquiring HPV, over 90% of women cleared after 2 years. Risk factors for persistence included increasing age, infection with more than one subtype and infection with high-risk types.

Table 3.2. Clinical manifestations and their associated human papillomavirus subtypes

	HPV subtype
Cutaneous warts	
Immunocompetent patients	
Common warts	2, 4
Verrucae plantaris/palmaris	1
Verrucae plana	3, 10, 28, 41
Butcher's warts	7
Immunocompromised patients	
Epidermodysplasia verruciformis	3, 5, 8, 9, 10, 12, 14, 15, 17, 19–25, 36–38, 47, 50
Iatrogenic	3, 5, 8, 9, 10, 12, 14, 15, 17, 19–25, 36–38
HIV	2, 6, 7, 11, 13, 16, 18, 32
Mucosal warts	
Anogenital	
Condyloma acuminata	6, 11
Penile cancer associated	16, 18
Vulvar cancer associated	16
Cervical cancer associated	6, 11, 16, 18, 31, 33, 35, 42–45, 51, 52, 56
Head and neck	
Oral and laryngeal	1, 2, 3,4 , 6, 7, 11, 13, 16, 18, 30–33, 35, 40, 52, 57
Conjunctival	6, 11

Although cervical disease in the woman is the most important sign of HPV, there are other manifestations, mainly in the form of condylomata acuminata. Infection of the cervix accounts for 70% of HPV disease, with much smaller numbers involving the vulva, vagina and anus.[68] Identification of condyloma is important to the patient because the disease can cause pain and psychological stress, although, perhaps more importantly, infection with one HPV type predisposes the patient to infection with others.

More studies are emerging that demonstrate HPV in male anogenital cancers. However, the data are not as solid when compared with female carcinoma. Squamous cell carcinoma (SCC) of the penis and the perineal area is a less common event than cervical cancer in the female population, with incidence rates in the USA and Europe estimated at 1 per 100 000.[69] This makes it difficult to conduct large studies. There appear to be multifactorial associations; circumcision and cigarette smoking are also confounding variables. Condylomata acuminata appear to be less common in the male population as well, although the disparity is not as striking as that of invasive carcinoma.[70] As previously mentioned for women, men can have a subclinical, carrier state of disease and promiscuity is the primary risk factor.[71,72] Implications have also been made that men are reservoirs for female infection and cervical cancer without actually manifesting disease themselves.[73] Nevertheless, HPVs have been observed in SCC in situ (as erythroplasia of Queyrat and bowenoid papulosis) with significant frequency. Usually, the HPVs are the high- and moderate-risk types and often mixed,

Table 3.3 Emerging cutaneous diseases associated with human papillomavirus

---

Fibroepithelial polyps (skin tags)
Seborrhoeic keratoses
Psoriasis
Basal cell carcinoma
Squamous cell carcinoma
Melanoma

---

especially when invasive disease is present.[69,74]

A contentious relationship has developed with regard to the presence of genital warts in children. Condylomata were once believed to be proof of sexual abuse, but molecular studies of HPV in patients have proved that perinatal passage and autoinoculation are possible acquisition sources.[75,76] HPV2 has been demonstrated in a number of cases.[75] Therefore, although sexual abuse should be excluded in every case, it should not be assumed until detailed information is obtained, in the form of history and physical examination of the patient (and family members, if possible) and, when warranted, detailed HPV typing.[77]

In addition to the diseases shown above and listed in Table 3.2, there are a number of dermatological conditions that have been loosely associated with HPV infection. Table 3.3 lists the emerging cutaneous diseases associated with HPV.

CONCLUSION

The vast numbers of HPVs produce numerous clinical manifestations. Although descriptions of condyloma can be traced from ancient times, our knowledge of the virus and its full scope of infectious properties are only now coming into focus. HPV is capable of produc-ing benign cutaneous verrucae on various locations of the body, with different subtypes favouring different areas, e.g. HPV1 shows specific predilection for the plantar surface of the foot. Completely different viruses infect mucosal epithelium and produce devastating, fatal consequences. Unfortunately, we know very little about how HPV gains entry into cells (i.e. its receptor) and, thus, why certain subtypes prefer different sites. It is easy to speculate that keratinization plays at least a part role – the mechanism of cornification in the integument is almost as diverse as the study of the papillomavirus itself. At this point, however, we have only a portion of the story.

As for the epidemiology of HPV, the murky waters are clearing. Cutaneous HPV is ubiquitous in the environment, and most people are exposed to the agent at an early age. The vast majority of individuals clear the infection with only mild manifestations or subclinical illness. There are disease states that predispose patients to more serious signs such as epidermodysplasia verruciformis and general cell-mediated immunodeficiencies. More emphasis in the epidemiological literature is understandably placed on mucosal disease. The primary mode of transmission of the mucosal HPVs is sexual, but other forms of intimate contact as well as parturition may be involved. HPV is now known to be the most common STD in the USA, and barrier devices such as condoms inhibit its passage. It is recommended that doctors reinforce the importance of these protective measures to their patients. Once exposed to mucosal HPV, the results for patients are similar to those with cutaneous infections: most will clear without sequelae. A small percentage (many more women than men) will progress from infection to transformation, developing frank invasive malignancies with poor prognoses. Risk factors for these events from the data gathered include promiscuity, subtype of HPV (especially types 16 and 18), multiple infections, and non-circumcision and cigarette smoking in men. The main focus of clinicians who treat patients with HPV is currently devoted to prevention and early detection as well as surgical excision, because there are few treatment options available currently for the patient who develops metastatic disease. Annual Pap smears for sexually active women, screening of sexual partners of HPV-infected patients for genital warts as well as other STDs, and the aggressive treatment of warts already present are all recommended proactive and counteractive measures. These steps have been already proved as cost-effective and life saving to innumerable individuals, and their emphasis will perpetuate this success.

REFERENCES

1. Carr J, Gyorfi T. Human papillomavirus epidemiology, transmission, and pathogenesis. *Clin Lab Med* 2000; **20**: 235–55.
2. Lorincz AT, Reid R, Jenson AB et al. Human papillomavirus infection of the cervix: relative risk associations of 15 common anogenital types. *Obstet Gynecol* 1992; **79**: 328–37.
3. Carter RL. *A Dictionary of Dermatologic Terms*, 4th edn. Baltimore: Williams & Wilkins, 1992: 341–2.
4. Oriel JD. Natural history of genital warts. *Br J Ven Dis* 1971; **47**: 1–13.
5. Bafverstedt B. Condylomata acuminata – past and present. *Acta Dermato-venereol* 1967; **47**: 376–81.
6. Wile UJ, Kingery LB. The etiology of common warts. *JAMA*, 1919; **73**: 970–3.
7. Koutsky LA, Galloway DA, Holmes KK. Epidemiology of genital human papillomavirus infection. *Epidemiol Rev* 1988; **10**: 122–63.
8. Voog E. Genital viral infections: Studies on human papillomavirus and Epstein–Barr virus. *Acta Dermato-venereol* 1996; **198**(suppl): 9–55.
9. Barrett TJ, Silbar JD, McGinley JP. Genital warts – a venereal disease. *JAMA* 1954; **154**: 333–4.
10. Beutner KR. Human papillomavirus and human disease. *Am J Med* 1997; **102**: 9–15.
11. Dianzani C, Calvieri S, Pierangeli A et al. The detection of human papillomavirus DNA in skin tags. *Br J Dermatol* 1998; **138**: 649–51.
12. Koutsky L. Epidemiology of genital human papillomavirus infection. *Am J Med* 1997; **102**: 3–8.
13. Melton JL, Rasmussen JE. Clinical manifestations of human papillomavirus infection in nongenital sites. *Dermatol Clin* 1991; **9**: 219–33.
14. Kilkenny M, Marks R. The descriptive epidemiology of warts in the community. *Austral J Dermatol* 1996; **37**: 80–6.
15. Stack PS. Pap smears. Still a reliable tool for cervical cancer. *Postgrad Med* 1997; **101**: 207–8.
16. Olsen AO, Killner J, Gjoen K, Magnus P. Seropositivity against HPV16 capsids: a better marker of past sexual behaviour than presence of HPV DNA. *Genitourin Med* 1997; **73**: 131–5.
17. Dillner J, Kallings I, Brihmer C et al. Seropositivities to human papillomavirus types 16, 18, or 33 capsids and to *Chlamydia trachomatis* are markers of sexual behavior. *J Infect Dis* 1996; **173**: 1394–8.
18. Andersson-Ellstrom A, Dillner J, Hagmar B et al. Comparison of development of serum antibodies to HPV 16 and HPV 33 and acquisition of cervical HPV DNA among sexually experienced and virginal young girls. *Sex Trans Dis* 1996; **23**: 234–8.
19. Jenson AB, Lancaster WD, Hartmann DP, Shaffer EL Jr. Frequency and distribution of papillomavirus structural antigens in verrucae, multiple papillomas, and condylomata of the oral cavity. *Am J Pathol* 1982; **107**: 212–18.
20. Jenson AB, Sommer S, Payling-Wright C et al. Human papillomavirus: Frequency and distribution in plantar and common warts. *Lab Investig* 1982; **47**: 491–7.

21. Jenson AB, Kurman RJ, Lancaster WD. Detection of papillomavirus common antigens in lesions of skin and mucosa. *Clin Dermatol* 1985; **3**: 56–63.

22. Zheng PS, Li SR, Iwasaka T et al. Simultaneous detection by consensus multiplex PCR of high- and low-risk and other types of human papillomavirus in clinical samples. *Gynecol Oncol* 1995; **58**: 179–83.

23. Stehr-Green PA, Hewer P, Meekin GE, Judd LE. The aetiology and risk factors for warts among poultry processing workers. *Int J Epidemiol* 1993; **22**: 294–8.

24. Johnson LW. Communal showers and the risk of plantar warts. *J Fam Pract* 1995; **40**: 136–8.

25. Popescu R, Popescu CM, Williams HC, Forsea D. The prevalence of skin conditions in Romanian school children. *Br J Dermatol* 1999; **140**: 891–6.

26. Kilkenny M, Merlin K, Young R, Marks R. The prevalence of common skin conditions in Australian school students: 1. Common, plane and plantar viral warts. *Br J Dermatol* 1998; **138**: 840–5.

27. Massing AM, Epstein WL. Natural history of warts. *Arch Dermatol* 1963; **87**: 306–10.

28. Moy R, Eliezri YD. Significance of human papillomavirus-induced squamous cell carcinoma to dermatologists. *Arch Dermatol* 1994; **130**: 235–8.

29. Clavel CE, Huu VP, Durlach AP et al. Mucosal oncogenic human papillomaviruses and extragenital Bowen disease. *Cancer* 1999; **86**: 282–7.

30. Uezato H, Hagiwara K, Ramuzi ST et al. Detection of human papillomavirus type 56 in extragenital Bowen's disease. *Acta Dermatovenereol* 1999; **79**: 311–13.

30a. Leigh IM, Glover MT. Skin cancer and warts in immunosuppressed renal transplant recipients. *Recent Results Cancer Res* 1995; **139**: 69–86.

31. Ferrandiz C, Fuente MJ, Ariza A et al. Detection and typing of human papillomavirus in skin lesions from renal transplant recipients and equivalent lesions from immunocompetent patients. *Arch Dermatol* 1998; **134**: 381–2.

32. Barr BB, Benton EC, McLaren K et al. Human papillomavirus infection and skin cancer in renal allograft recipients. *Lancet* 1989; **i**: 124–9.

33. Smith SE, Davis IC, Leshin B et al. Absence of human papillomavirus in squamous cell carcinomas from nongenital skin from immunocompromised renal transplant patients. *Arch Dermatol* 1993; **129**: 1285–8.

34. Harwood CA, Surentheran T, McGregor JM et al. Human papillomavirus infection and non-melanoma skin cancer in immunosuppressed and immunocompetent individuals. *J Med Virol* 2000; **61**: 289–97.

35. Chopra KF, Tyring SK. The impact of the human immunodeficiency virus on the human papillomavirus epidemic. *Arch Dermatol* 1997; **133**: 629–33.

36. Greenspan D, de Villiers EM, Greenspan JS et al. Unusual HPV types in oral warts in association with HIV infection. *J Oral Pathol* 1988; **17**: 482–7.

37. Trottier AM, Coutlee F, Leduc R. Human immunodeficiency virus infection is a major risk factor for detection of human papillomavirus DNA in esophageal brushings. *Clin Infect Dis* 1997; **24**: 565–9.

38. Ramoz N, Rueda LA, Bouadjar B et al. A susceptibility locus for epidermodysplasia verruciformis, an abnormal predisposition to infection with the oncogenic human papillomavirus type 5, maps to chromosome 7qter in a region containing the psoriasis locus. *J Invest Dermatol* 1999; **112**: 259–63.

39. Ramoz N, Taieb A, Rueda LA et al. Evidence for a nonallelic heterogeneity of epidermodysplasia verruciformis with two susceptibility loci mapped to chromosome regions 2p21–p24 and 17q25. *J Invest Dermatol* 2000; **114**: 1148–53.

40. Majewski S, Skopinska-Rozewska E, Jablonska S et al. Partial defects of cell-mediated immunity in patients with epider-

modysplasia verruciformis. *J Am Acad Dermatol* 1986; **15**: 966–73.

41. Orth G. Epidermodysplasia verruciformis: a model for understanding the oncogenicity of human papillomaviruses. *Ciba Foundation Symposium* 1986; **120**: 157–74.

42. Roden BS, Lowy DR, Schiller JT. Papillomavirus is resistant to desiccation. *J Infect Dis* 1997; **176**: 1076–9.

43. De Villiers EM, Weidauer H, Otto H, zur Hausen H. Papillomavirus DNA in human tongue carcinomas. *Int J Cancer* 1985; **36**: 575–8.

44. Atula S, Auvinen E, Grenman R, Syrjanen S. Human papillomavirus and Epstein–Barr virus in epithelial carcinomas of the head and neck region. *Anticancer Res* 1997; **17**: 4427–34.

45. Terai M, Takagi M, Matsukura T, Sata T. Oral wart associated with human papillomavirus type 2. *J Oral Pathol Med* 1999; **28**: 137–40.

46. Maitland NJ, Cox MF, Lynas C et al. Detection of human papillomavirus DNA in biopsies of human oral tissue. *Br J Cancer* 1987; **56**: 245–50.

47. Jalal H, Sanders CM, Prime SS et al. Detection of human papillomavirus type 16 DNA in oral squames from normal young adults. *J Oral Pathol Med* 1992; **21**: 465–70.

48. Kellokoski JK, Syrjanen SM, Chang F. Southern blot hybridization and PCR in detection of oral human papillomavirus infections in women with genital HPV infections. *J Oral Pathol Med* 1992; **21**: 459–64.

49. Pfister H, Hettich I, Runne U et al. Characterization of human papillomavirus type 13 from focal epithelial hyperplasia Heck lesions. *J Virol* 1983; **47**: 363–6.

50. McDonnell PJ, McDonnell JM, Kessis T et al. Detection of human papillomavirus type 6/11 DNA in conjunctival papillomas by in situ hybridization with radioactive probes. *Hum Pathol* 1987; **18**: 1115–19.

51. Centers for Disease Control and Prevention web site, www.cdc.gov/nchstp/od/news/ RevBrochure1pdfhpv.htm (8 October, 2001).

52. Cates W. Estimates of the incidence and prevalence of sexually transmitted diseases in the United States. *Sex Trans Dis* 1999; **26** (suppl 4): 2–7.

53. Centers for Disease Control and Prevention web site, www.cdc.gov/nchstp/od/news/ RevBrochure1pdfcloselookhpv.htm (8 October, 2001).

54. Stone KM. Human papillomavirus infection and genital warts: Update on epidemiology and treatment. *Clin Infect Dis* 1995; **20**(suppl 1): 91–7.

55. Dillner J, Meijer CJ, von Krogh G, Horenblas S. Epidemiology of human papillomavirus infection. *Scand J Urol Nephrol* 2000; **205** (suppl):194–200.

56. Ferenczy A, Bergeron C, Richart RM. Human papillomavirus DNA in fomites on objects used for the management of patients with genital human papillomavirus infections. *Obstet Gynecol* 1989; **74**: 950–4.

57. Gutman LT, Herman-Giddens ME, Phelps WC. Transmission of human genital papillomavirus disease: Comparison of data from adults and children. *Pediatrics* 1993; **91**: 31–8.

58. Fairley CK, Gay NJ, Forbes A et al. Hand–genital transmission of genital warts? An analysis of prevalence data. *Epidemiol Infect* 1995; **115**: 169–76.

59. Zur Hausen H. Condylomata acuminata and human genital cancer. *Cancer Res* 1976; **36**: 794.

60. Melchers WJ, Bakkers JM, Wang J et al. Short fragment polymerase chain reaction reverse hybridization line probe assay to detect and genotype a broad spectrum of human papillomavirus types. *Am J Pathol* 1999; **155**: 1473–8.

61. Bosch FX, Manos MM, Munoz N et al. Prevalence of human papillomavirus in cervical cancer: a worldwide perspective. *J Natl Cancer Inst* 1995; **87**: 796–802.

62. Jamison JH, Kaplan DW, Hamman R et al. Spectrum of genital human papillomavirus infection in a female adolescent population. *Sex Trans Dis* 1995; **22**: 236–43.

63. Ho GY, Bierman R, Beardsley NP et al.

Natural history of cervicovaginal papillomavirus infection in young women. *N Engl J Med* 1998; **338**: 423–8.

64. Azocar J, Abad SM, Acosta H et al. Prevalence of cervical dysplasia and HPV infection according to sexual behavior. *Int J Cancer* 1990; **45**: 622–5.

65. Negrini BP, Schiffman MH, Kurman RJ et al. Oral contraceptive use, human papillomavirus infection, and risk of early cytological abnormalities of the cervix. *Cancer Res* 1990; **50**: 4670–5.

66. Slattery ML, Overall JC, Abbott TM et al. Sexual activity, contraception, genital infections, and cervical cancer: Support for a sexually transmitted disease hypothesis. *Am J Epidemiol* 1989; **130**: 248–58.

67. Andersson-Ellstrom A, Dillner J, Hagmar B et al. No serological evidence for non-sexual spread of HPV 16. *Lancet* 1994; **344**: 1435.

68. Ferenczy A. Epidemiology and clinical pathophysiology of condylomata acuminata. *Am J Obstet Gynecol* 1995; **172**: 1331–9.

69. Griffiths TR, Mellon JK. Human papillomavirus and urological tumours: I. Basic science and role in penile cancer. *BJU Int* 1999; **84**: 579–86.

70. Persson G, Andersson K, Krantz I. Symptomatic genital papillomavirus infection in a community. *Acta Obstet Gynaecol Scand* 1996; **75**: 287–90.

71. Grussendorf-Conen EI, De Villiers EM, Gissmann L. Human papillomavirus genomes in penile smears of healthy men. *Lancet*, 1986; **ii**: 1092.

72. Hippelainen M, Syrjanen S, Hippelainen M et al. Prevalence and risk factors of genital human papillomavirus infections in healthy males: A study of Finnish conscripts. *Sex Transmit Dis* 1993; **20**: 321–8.

73. Bosch FX, Castellsague X, Munoz N et al. Male sexual behavior and human papillomavirus DNA: Key risk factors for cervical cancer in Spain. *J Natl Cancer Inst* 1996; **88**: 1060–7.

74. Park KC, Kim KH, Youn SW et al. Heterogeity of human papillomavirus DNA in a patient with bowenoid papulosis that progressed to squamous cell carcinoma. *Br J Dermatol* 1998; **139**: 1087–91.

75. Armstrong DK, Handley JM. Anogenital warts in children: pathogenesis, HPV typing and management. *Int J STD AIDS* 1997; **8**: 78–81.

76. Hammerschlag MR. Sexually transmitted diseases in sexually abused children: medical and legal implications. *Sex Transm Infect* 1998; **74**: 167–74.

77. Schachner L, Hankin DE. Assessing child abuse in childhood condyloma acuminatum. *J Am Acad Dermatol* 1985; **12**: 157–60.

4 Clinical manifestations

Amy Helms and Robert T Brodell

Cutaneous lesions • Mucocutaneous lesions • Conclusion • References

Almost everyone has either had a wart or knows someone who has had one. Human papillomaviruses (HPVs) are involved in the development of a range of diseases, from common warts to the rare epidermodysplasia verruciformis (EV).[1,2] Although they are all caused by HPV infection, warts appear in many locations and show a variety of shapes and sizes.[3] Still, the lesions have a characteristic appearance that often makes the diagnosis obvious to both the patient and the physician. It is the purpose of this chapter to distill the essence of these characteristics so that, with a little experience, the diagnosis of warts can be based primarily on their clinical features.

The Roman word for a wart was verruca, which meant little hill or eminence. The adjective 'verrucous' describes the multitude of tiny surface projections, which is the hallmark of clinical skin infection with HPV. These clinical findings are histopathologically reflected as hyperplasia or thickening of the epidermis, papillomatosis or microscopic projections of the epithelium, and hyperkeratosis. Warts can occur on keratinized epithelium and on mucosal surfaces of the mouth, esophagus, vagina, anus, larynx, trachea, and conjunctiva.

The clinical characteristics of warts depend in part on the type of HPV causing the infection. The location, age of the lesion, environmental factors, and internal immune factors also play a role. Warts may be small and flat, or large and quite elevated, even 'cauliflower like'. They may grow as a tiny solitary papule or coalesce and form extensive plaques.

Although a variety of methods has been used to classify warts based on their appearance, location, and viral type, no method has been universally accepted. We have modified the classification scheme of Bunney that is based on viral type and focused on the morphology of these lesions (Table 4.1). This scheme separates warts into two major categories: cutaneous and mucocutaneous.

CUTANEOUS LESIONS

Common warts (*verruca vulgaris*)

The common wart is a hyperkeratotic papilloma typically located on the hands, fingers, or soles of the feet. Common warts are seen primarily in children and teenagers. In toddlers, common warts may also be found on genital or perigenital skin.[6–8] These verrucous papules are usually 1–4 mm in diameter, thin or thick, with a rough, gray, tan, or brown surface that may lead to fissuring and tenderness,

Table 4.1 A system of classification utilizing location, morphology, and human papillomavirus (HPV) types.

Group	Type of lesion	Type of HPV
Cutaneous	Common warts:	2, 4, 7, 27, 29
	• Typical	2, 4, 7
	• Mosaic	2
	• Papillomatous	2, 4, 7
	• Endophytic	4
	Deep plantar (myrmecia)	1
	Flat warts	3, 10, 28, 49
Mucocutaneous	Genital warts:	6, 11, 16, 18, 42
	• Condyloma acuminata	6, 11
	• Flat condyloma	16, 18
	Bowenoid papulosis	16, 55

especially when they are large and thick (Figure 4.1). Warts are highly vascular lesions and often bleed profusely when bumped. Blood vessels in the dermal papillae extend close to the surface of the wart and are responsible for this feature. Tiny black dots are also frequently seen in common warts. Although often referred to as 'seeds' by patients, they are in fact tiny thrombosed capillaries (Figure 4.2).[4] Another common feature can be used to distinguish warts from calluses. Warts disrupt the dermatoglyphics or 'fingerprint' lines, whereas in calluses these lines extend from the surrounding normal skin in an uninterrupted fashion over the surface of the lesion.[9]

Common warts may spread by autoinoculation. For this reason, satellite lesions are often present in the vicinity of a wart. In addition, scalloping can be seen at the edge of a large wart and represents incorporation of sites of autoinoculation in adjacent skin as the wart expands (Figures 4.3 and 4.4). Finally, warts are often present on two skin surfaces that touch when the body is at rest. Of course, they can be found anywhere on the body.

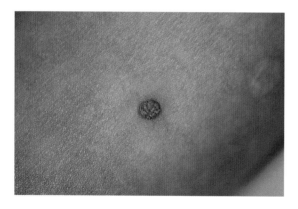

Figure 4.1
A 5-mm diameter wart present on the lateral upper arm. It demonstrates typical verrucous surface projections.

Mosaic warts

Multiple grouped warts that look like a single verrucous plaque are referred to as a mosaic wart.[10] Satellite lesions are also commonly seen outside the areas of coalescent plaque.

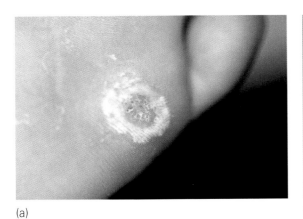

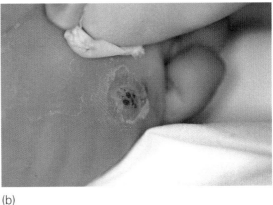

(a)   (b)

Figure 4.2
(a) A wart is present on the left foot. It shows verrucous surface features, thrombosed capillaries, and focal crusting. (b) After paring there is pinpoint bleeding.

Figure 4.3
Multiple warts of diameter 1–4 mm are found on the right knee. The larger lesions show scalloped edges representing a coalescence of smaller warts. Topical anesthesia with eutectic mixture of local anesthetics (EMLA) under occlusion hydrated the lesions, leading to their white color.

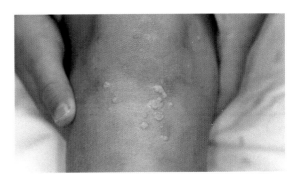

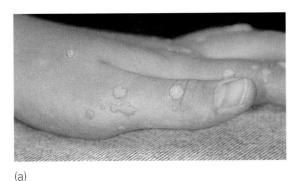

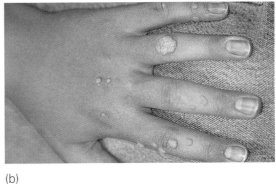

(a)   (b)

Figure 4.4
(a) Multiple warts of diameter 1–16 mm on the right thumb demonstrating verrucous surface features and white scale. The larger lesions represent a coalescence of smaller warts. (b) Dozens of similar warts on the rest of this patient's hand emphasize the difficulty in treating patients with multiple lesions.

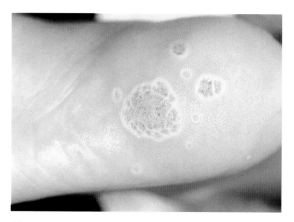

Figure 4.5
A mosaic wart of 25-mm diameter present on the plantar surface of the left heel with several satellite lesions. Thrombosed capillaries and a moth-eaten appearance are noted.

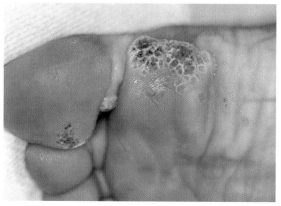

Figure 4.6
This large mosaic wart has several satellite lesions and shows crusting. 'Black dots' represent thrombosed capillaries.

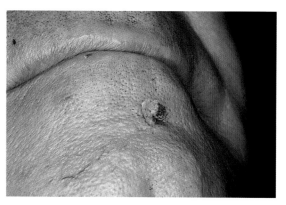

Figure 4.7
A pedunculated wart of 4-mm diameter on the chin, which is constantly irritated and bleeds profusely when nicked while shaving.

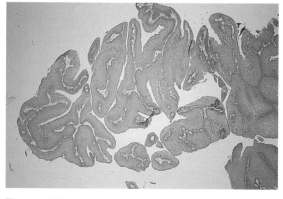

Figure 4.8
Histopathology of a papillomatous wart shows acanthosis and papillomatosis, with finger-like projections that are cut in cross-section. The presence of telangiectasias within the papillary dermal projections correlates with the tendency for these lesions to bleed when traumatized. (Magnification × 40; stained with hematoxylin and eosin (H&E.)

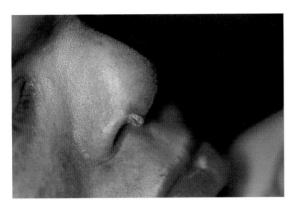

Figure 4.9
This crusted papillomatous lesion at the opening to the left nares is constantly irritated and often bled on the slightest trauma.

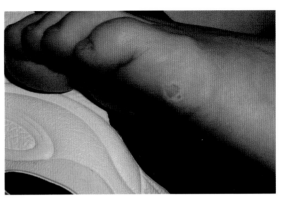

Figure 4.10
Small hyperkeratotic punctate depressions are noted at the base of this left little toe.

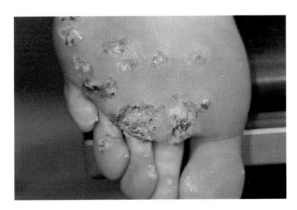

Figure 4.11
Numerous thick, keratotic, crusted lesions are present on the sole of the foot. Black dots represent thrombosed capillaries within dermal papillae.

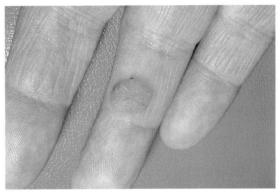

Figure 4.12
This verrucous lesion has a collarette margin, which interrupts the dermatoglyphs on the finger.

They may be a few millimeters to several centimeters in diameter. Mosaic warts are commonly seen on the palms and soles (Figure 4.5). They can be quite thick and are often tender, especially when on the soles because of the pressure focused on these sites during ambulation. Attempts to pare the warts down often demonstrate thrombosed capillaries or cause pinpoint bleeding when vessels of the dermal papillae are transected (Figure 4.6).

Papillomatous warts

Viral growths may show predominantly vertical growth, resulting in a long, thin, filiform lesion or a pedunculated papule. Typical verrucous surface changes are also seen in these lesions. They are usually 2–4 mm in diameter, but can be are larger. As they are elevated from the surrounding skin, they are easily traumatized, bleed profusely, and often appear crusted (Figures 4.7–4.9).

Endophytic warts

Small, well-defined punctate depressions 1–2 mm in size are often seen on the palms or soles in early evolving verrucae. These may occur singly or in clusters. They may evolve into large mosaic warts (Figure 4.10).

Plantar and palmar warts (*verruca plantaris* and *palmaris*)

Typically found on the plantar and palmar surfaces, these thickened endophytic papules are extremely painful. They are often grouped at the pressure points on the ball of the foot (Figure 4.11).[11,12] These lesions, like common

warts, interrupt the normal skin lines or dermatoglyphs (Figures 4.12 and 4.13). They may be small, single lesions or coalesce to form large thick plaques 1–2 cm or more in size (Figure 4.14).

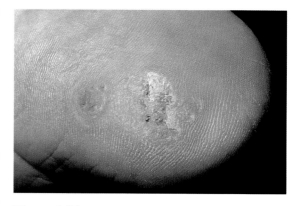

Figure 4.13
These keratotic warts interrupt the dermatoglyphs on the plantar surface of the heel. Focal crusting and black dots are also noted.

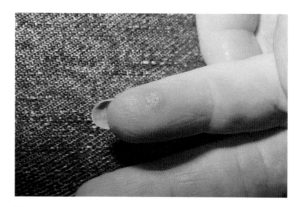

Figure 4.14
A scaling, verrucous papule 5-mm diameter is present on the right fifth finger. Close examination demonstrates a coalescence of smaller warts, causing a scalloped edge. The keratotic appearance of this lesion is typical of palmar and plantar warts.

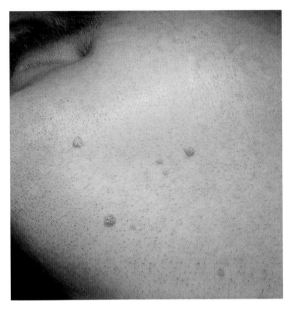

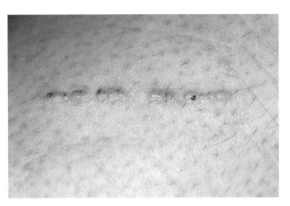

Figure 4.17
A dozen flat warts of diameter 1–1.5 mm present in a linear array on the left leg. The patient remembers excoriating warts at this site while shaving.

Figure 4.15
Flat warts on the neck in the beard area of a man. These are small and usually skin colored to slightly tan and pink, although they may be dark brown in darkly pigmented patients.

Flat warts (*verruca plana*)

Also referred to as juvenile warts, these small, flat-topped lesions occur most often on the hands and faces of children. In adults they are typically found on the neck, wrists, face, knees, hands, and foreheads (Figure 4.15). They may be misdiagnosed as acne vulgaris when on the face and neck (Figure 4.16). Flat warts are usually 1–4 mm in diameter and flesh colored. They may show koebnerization, or linear spread secondary to trauma, and are frequently spread by shaving the beard area of men or legs of women (Figure 4.17).

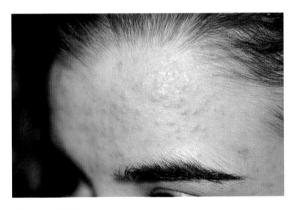

Figure 4.16
Numerous flat warts on the forehead can easily be mistaken for acne vulgaris if not examined carefully.

MUCOCUTANEOUS LESIONS

Genital warts (*condyloma acuminatum*)

Genital warts are the most common sexually transmitted disease and are frequently referred to as 'venereal' warts.[10,13,14] About a million

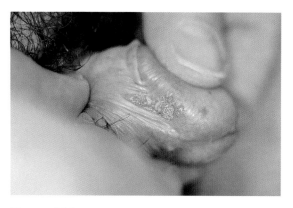

Figure 4.18
An 8 mm × 3 mm patch of coalescent warts of various sizes present in a moist area under the foreskin at the corona of the penis. Verrucous surface features are also noted.

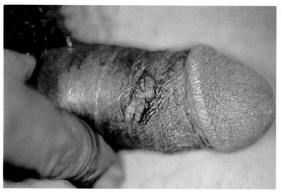

Figure 4.19
Confluent warts form a 6 mm × 10 mm plaque on the penis. Modest hyperpigmentation is also noted compared with the surrounding skin.

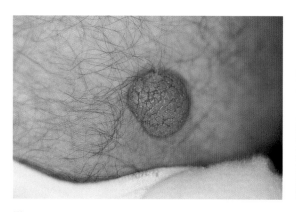

Figure 4.20
A 1-cm pink sessile wart present on the abdomen. It shows verrucous surface features with pinpoint foci of crusting.

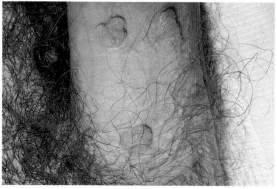

Figure 4.21
Several genital warts present on the shaft of the penis. These lesions demonstrate subtle 'verrucous' surface features, and the confluence of smaller warts, which lead to scalloping of the edges of evolving lesions.

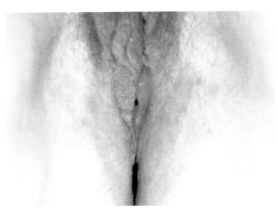

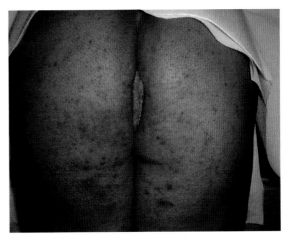

(a)

Figure 4.22
A 2 cm × 1 cm finely papillomatous mass present on the left labia minora. Smaller pinpoint satellite lesions are also noted.

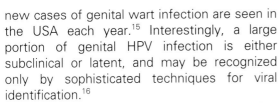

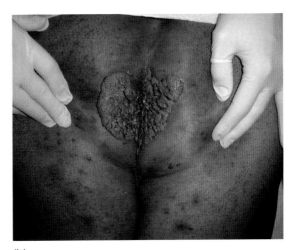

(b)

Figure 4.23
(a) Cauliflower-like perianal warts which, at first glance, appear to be a largely cosmetic problem. (b) The same perianal wart is fully exposed, demonstrating moistness and maceration, which correlate with a history of itching and burning. Residual stool is also noted and this highlights the difficulty patients experience maintaining adequate hygiene.

new cases of genital wart infection are seen in the USA each year.[15] Interestingly, a large portion of genital HPV infection is either subclinical or latent, and may be recognized only by sophisticated techniques for viral identification.[16]

Genital warts are small, pointed papules that are usually 2–5 mm in diameter, but they may coalesce and measure several centimeters in diameter and height (Figures 4.18 and 4.19). They are typically gray, skin colored, pink, or brown (Figure 4.20). Generally speaking, genital warts are found in the anogenital areas of both men and women. Typically, they are present in men on the shaft of the penis, coronal sulcus, prepuce, frenulum, and anus (Figure 4.21). In women, genital warts inhabit the mucosal surfaces of the vulva, the perineum, and the anus (Figures 4.22 and 4.23). Large 'cauliflower-like' masses may develop in moist, occluded areas such as the perianal skin, vulva, and inguinal folds (Figures 4.24 and 4.25).

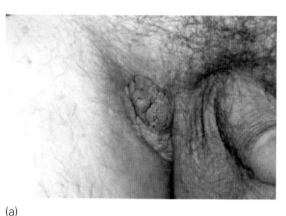
(a)

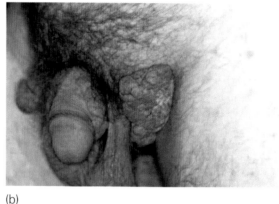
(b)

Figure 4.24
(a) A 5 cm × 3 cm 'cauliflower-like' mass present in the right inguinal fold. Verrucous surface features and focal crusting are noted. (b) The left inguinal fold demonstrates a similar mass.

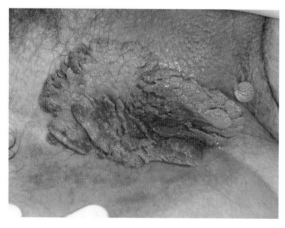

Figure 4.25
A large moist, macerated, inflamed mass of wart present within the inguinal fold.

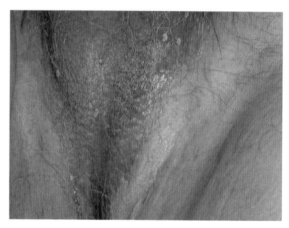

Figure 4.26
Flat-topped warts on the vulva measure 0.5–1.0 mm in diameter.

Flat condylomata

Warts appearing in the urethra, the perianal areas, and sometimes on the scrotum and genitalia may be very small and have a flat rather than a verrucous surface. These do not tend to grow into cauliflower-like clusters and usually remain only 1–3 mm in size (Figures 4.26 and 4.27).

Bowenoid papulosis

These lesions are characterized by small, smooth, flat papules, which may be discrete or sometimes grouped on the penis. The lesions were initially described on the glans or shaft and may be translucent to dusky red or hyperpigmented. These features are often indistinguishable from other HPV-induced genital

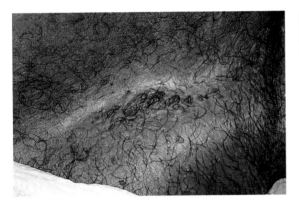

Figure 4.27
Hyperpigmented flat-topped warts present on the thigh and within the groin where they become confluent.

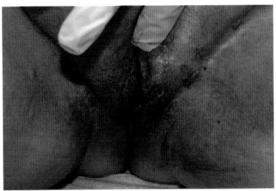

Figure 4.28
Bowenoid papules seen on the external genitalia and perineal skin. They are typically darker than the normal skin color.

warts, although on biopsy they show keratinocyte atypia with a 'shot-gunned' appearance scattered throughout the epidermis. It has, therefore, been referred to as penile squamous cell carcinoma *in situ*, although these lesions tend to be slow growing and evolve in a similar fashion to genital warts rather than carcinoma.[17] Similar clinical and histologic findings have been described in women, affecting the labia, perineum, or inguinal folds (Figure 4.28).[18]

Special cases

Warts can be affected by external factors such as frictional forces and trauma, which often cause these lesions to become irritated (Figure 4.29). Also, warts may become infected leading to redness, pain, heat, and lymphangitis (Figure 4.30). Periungual and subungual warts are lesions that occur under and around the fingernails and toenails (Figures 4.31–4.33). A particularly unusual distribution of warts has been described within the black dye of tattoos. The dye may decrease local immune responses and permit these warts to thrive,

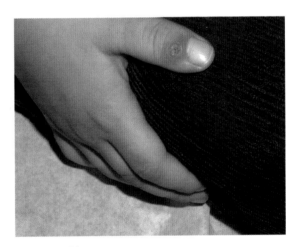

Figure 4.29
This crusted 9-mm wart on the right thumb became tender 3 days after being excoriated.

while they are suppressed in the adjacent non-tattooed skin (Figure 4.34).[19] Warts often develop a thick cap of hyperkeratosis, which elongates slowly over the years and can result in a cutaneous horn (Figure 4.35). Cutaneous horns can also occur overlying actinic keratosis and squamous cell carcinoma.

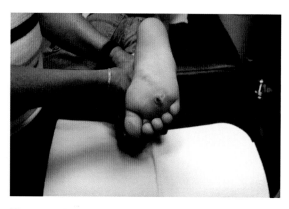

Figure 4.30
A tender 9 mm × 9 mm wart on the sole of the left foot developed a lymphangitic streak extending proximally on the instep.

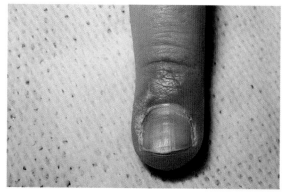

Figure 4.31
A 6 mm × 2 mm diameter periungual wart involved the lateral nailfold. It shows verrucous surface features and thrombosed capillaries.

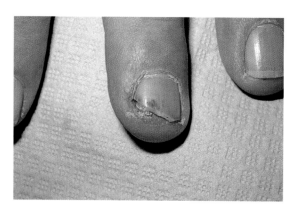

Figure 4.32
A 4 mm × 4 mm subungual wart is visible at the free edge of the nail. Onycholysis of the distal nail corresponds to more proximal involvement.

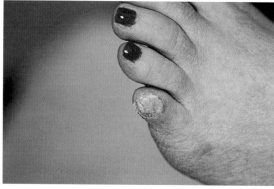

Figure 4.33
This subungual wart led to loss of the overlying nail, and involves the entire nail bed of the right little toe. Squamous cell carcinoma would also have to be considered in a wart with this type of presentation.

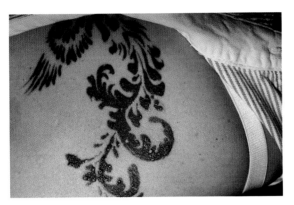

Figure 4.34
Scattered flat warts are present within the black dye of this tattoo. There were only a few warts on normal skin outside the tattooed area, suggesting that the dye may have adversely affected local immune surveillance.

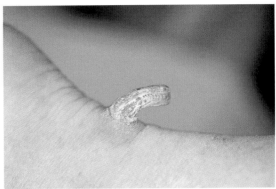

Figure 4.35
This curled cutaneous horn measuring 3 mm × 3 mm × 18 mm was present over the Achilles' tendon. It lengthened slowly over a period of 6 months. Pathology showed a viral wart beneath the cutaneous horn.

CONCLUSION

Warts may present with lesions of many sizes, shapes, colors, and configurations on various parts of the body. The diagnosis is usually based on clinical manifestations. On occasion, variations in morphologic features as well as erythema, crusting, and marked hyperkeratosis may make differentiation from actinic keratoses or squamous cell carcinomas difficult. In this case a biopsy may be necessary to confirm the diagnosis.

REFERENCES

1. Beutner KR, Tyring S. Human papillomavirus and human disease. *Am J Med* 1997; **102**: 9–15.
2. Tyring SK. Human papillomavirus infections: epidemiology, pathogenesis, and host immune response. *J Am Acad Dermatol* 2000; **43**: 518–26.
3. Weston WL, Lane AT, Morelli JG. *Color Textbook of Pediatric Dermatology*, 2nd edn. St Louis: Mosby, 1996: 121–30.
4. Freedberg IM, Eisen AZ, Wolff K et al. *Dermatology in General Medicine*, 5th edn. New York: McGraw-Hill, 1999.
5. Bunney MH, Benton C, Cubie H. *Viral Warts: Biology and Treatment*, 2nd edn. Oxford: Oxford University Press, 1992.
6. Gutman LT. Transmission of human genital papillomavirus disease: comparison data for adults and children. *Pediatrics* 1993; **91**: 31.
7. Handley JM, Maw RD, Bingham EA et al. Anogenital warts in children. *Clin Exp Dermatol* 1993; **18**: 241.
8. Hurwitz S. Anogenital warts and sexual abuse in children: a perspective. *Fitzpatrick's J Clin Dermatol* 1994; Mar/Apr: 38.
9. Cohen BA. *Atlas of Pediatric Dermatology*. London: Wolfe, 1993: 5.5–5.7.
10. Domonkos AN, Arnold HL, Odom RB. *Andrew's Diseases of the Skin*, 7th edn. Philadelphia: WB Saunders Co., 1982.
11. Farmer ER, Hood AF. *Pathology of the Skin*, 2nd edn. New York: McGraw-Hill, 1990.

12. Rook A, Wilkinson DS, Ebling FJG. *Textbook of Dermatology*, Vol 1. Philadelphia: FA Davis Co., 1968.
13. Maw R, von Krogh G. The management of anal warts. *BMJ* 2000; **321**: 910–11.
14. Moresi JM, Herbert CR, Cohen BA. Treatment of anogenital warts in children with topical 0.05% Podofilox gel and 5% Imiquimod cream. *Pediatr Dermatol* 2001; **18**: 448–52.
15. Obalek S, Jablonska S, Orth G. Anogenital warts in children. *Clin Dermatol* 1997; **15**: 369–76.
16. Sawchuk WS. Ancillary diagnostic tests for detection of human papillomavirus infection. *Dermatol Clin* 1991; **9**: 277.
17. Stone MS, Lynch PJ. Viral warts. In: Sams WM Jr, Lynch PJ, eds. *Principles and Practice in Dermatology*, 2nd edn. New York: Churchill Livingstone, 1996: 127–35.
18. Jablonska S, Majewski S. Human papillomavirus infection in women. *Clin Dermatol* 1997; **15**: 67–79.
19. Miller DM, Brodell RT. Verruca restricted to the areas of black dye within a tattoo. *Arch Dermatol* 1994; **130**: 1453–4.

Part II
Home therapies

5 Acids in the treatment of viral warts

Angeline F Lim, Sanjay Sheth and Robert T Brodell

Historical aspects • Classification • Basic science • Clinical studies • Favored treatment methodology • Adverse effects • Cost–benefit considerations • Case reports • References

As most people will have been afflicted with at least one wart at some point during their lives, and there is little urgency for immediate clearing, it is no surprise that there is an entire industry catering to the public demand for home wart treatments.

Americans spend more than $US45 million annually on over-the-counter wart products.[1] Despite the broad array of formulations available, most home treatments rely on an acid as their active ingredient, most commonly salicylic acid. For some over-the-counter treatments, salicylic acid is combined with lactic acid. There are other caustic agents available to the physician for treatment in the surgery, including monochloroacetic acid (MCAA), dichloroacetic acid (DCAA) and trichloroacetic acid (TCAA). In this chapter, we review the treatment of warts with various types of acids, emphasizing primarily home treatments.

HISTORICAL ASPECTS

Salicylic acid and its derivatives have been used for centuries in the treatment of many common ailments. The Egyptians were the first to use salicylic acid and this was continued through the Greek civilization, where Hippocrates documented the use of a substance found in willow bark for the treatment of headaches and fevers. In America, Native American medicine men used willow bark in a similar manner. In 1838, Johan Andreas Buchner became the first person to isolate salicylic acid as the active compound in willow bark.[2] In response to its unpleasant side effects, a German chemist named Felix Hoffmann modified salicylic acid into acetylsalicylic acid or aspirin in the 1890s. In 1923, prescriptions for a salicylic acid and lactic acid combination, similar to the formulations available for home treatment today, were first used in the treatment of warts.[3]

CLASSIFICATION

Acids used in the home treatment of warts are available in a variety of strengths and bases. The most commonly used product is salicylic acid, available in variable strengths in the form of creams, gels, lotions, ointments, plasters and topical solutions, e.g. most over-the-counter solutions have concentrations of 17% salicylic acid (Occlusal-HP) whereas plasters can have as much as 40% (Clear Away). It may also be formulated with other additives such as lactic acid (Duofilm). The scientific literature has reported the use of salicylic acid in strengths up to 70% in clinical studies, which may be compounded by many pharmacists.[4] MCAA, DCAA and TCAA are generally used as a physician-applied treatment for use in the surgery.

BASIC SCIENCE

There is general agreement about the mechanism for salicylic acid in the treatment for warts. It is a keratolytic agent, which disrupts intercellular cohesiveness, causing desquamation of the human papillomavirus (HPV)-infected epidermal cells.[5] It may also cause triggering of a beneficial immune response, leading to regression.[6]

Other types of acids, including TCAA, work in a similar manner and because of their potency can be considered a form of chemical cautery.[7] TCAA non-specifically hydrolyses cellular proteins, leading to inflammation and cell death of both virally infected and normal cells.[8] In addition, it also provokes a humoral immune response that complements and strengthens the mechanochemical effects.[9]

CLINICAL STUDIES

In 2001 Sterling et al[6] set forth guidelines for the management of cutaneous warts. They considered salicylic acid to be first-line therapy for small warts. Available over the counter for home therapy, it is certainly convenient, although there have been relatively few placebo-controlled trials for accurate determination of its efficacy in the treatment of warts. Response rates for this modality are highly variable, ranging from 40% to 84%, with an average of 61%.[10] One of the earliest studies, conducted by Bunney in 1973,[11] found no difference in efficacy between daily application of 5% 5-fluorouracil in dimethyl sulphoxide and

a paint containing 16.7% salicylic acid and 16.7% lactic acid in four parts of flexible collodion (Duofilm) in the treatment of plantar warts (47–53% clearing). Later in the two-centre Edinburgh and Dundee trial, no statistical difference was found between the cure rate for hand warts treated with liquid nitrogen (69%) and those treated with equal parts of salicylic acid and lactic acid in four parts of flexible collodion (69%).[3] In another study, a combination of 12% salicylic acid, a small amount of lactic acid and a collodion gel (Salactac) applied nightly cured or markedly improved common warts in 75% of patients.[12] In warts treated with 15% salicylic acid in a karaya gum patch (TRANS-VER-SAL system), a 69% cure rate was found for verruca vulgaris.[13] This treatment also proved to be very safe and convenient.

A 60% cure rate was reported after 6 weeks of treatment with 21% salicylic acid polymeric matrix delivery system (Transplantar).[14] Topical salicylic acid solutions, such as the high-potency (26%) salicylic acid in a novel polyacrylic vehicle (Occlusal-HP), have an improvement or cure rate of 81% after only 2 weeks of treatment.[15] Unfortunately, those topicals with more than 17% salicylic acid have been removed from the US market pending further study of safety and efficacy. Most recently, van Brederode and Engel[4] reported an 89.2% resolution rate using a novel combination of weekly cryotherapy with Verruca-freeze and daily topical 70% salicylic acid with a mean treatment time of 7.6 weeks and an average of just 4.05 applications of Verruca-freeze.[4]

Treatment with salicylic acid is classified as level 1 based on the strength of evidence using our modified Evidence-based Medicine System (see Chapter 19). Its use is supported by good evidence from well-designed randomized controlled trials with narrow confidence intervals.[3,4,10–15] Larger randomized placebo controlled studies would be helpful to fully elevate this treatment method.

There is also significant variation in the clinical success rates for the other types of acid used in treating warts. Once-weekly treatments with 95% TCAA showed 70–81% response rates with similar efficacy; when compared with cryotherapy. In these studies, both TCAA and cryotherapy also showed similar adverse effects in the treatment of genital warts.[17–19] Higher success rates (90%) for MCAA were reported by Dagnall[20] but have not been replicated by others. A 66% cure rate using various formulations of MCAA was achieved by both Dutta[21] and Steele and Irwin[9] in separate trials. Treatment with MCAA, DCAA and TCAA is classified as level IIa based on our Modified Evidence-based Medicine System (see Chapter 19).

FAVORED TREATMENT METHODOLOGY (Table 5.1)

Salicylic acid is an excellent first-line home treatment for plane warts on the face, as well as for small warts on the hands and feet.[6] Many clinicians prefer to use collodion gels because of their ease of application and acceptability by patients. They can be applied quickly and accurately to the wart while drying quickly to form a transparent film.[8,22,23]

The protocol used by the authors is as follows: first, any film from previous treatments should be peeled off, and the wart mechanically débrided of any excess keratotic material. This may be achieved by using sandpaper, an emery board, pumis stone or nail file. This is done to ensure that the medication will destroy deeper layers of the wart. In addition, salicylic acid is combined with cantharidin, liquid nitrogen and other methods available in the surgery; efforts to débride the wart at home decrease the need for débridement at the surgery using a scalpel where bleeding can interfere with the treatment. Next, the patient should soak the area around the wart in warm water for several minutes and then pat the area dry. An applicator is used to apply the salicylic acid product to the wart, avoiding surrounding normal skin. The area may be covered with occlusive tape, especially in high-pressure areas such as the plantar surface of the foot or to prevent clothing from rubbing off the salicylic acid. The patient should repeat this process every night until the wart clears or for 6 weeks; 2- to 3-day 'holidays' from acid application may be taken if tenderness becomes a problem. This treatment protocol (Table 5.2) can be extended for weeks or months as needed for persistent warts, so long as progress is reported.[24] The treatment protocol is similar for other formulations of salicylic acid. When using salicylic acid patches, the patches should be trimmed to fit

Table 5.1 Acid treatment methodology

Type of acid	Strength (%)		No. of treatments/week
	OTC	Office	
Salicyclic acid	< 17	< 70	7 (OTC)1 (Office)
MCAA, DCAA, TCAA	NA	50–95	1

DCAA, dichloroacetic acid; MCAA, monochloroacetic acid; OTC, over the counter; TCAA, trichloroacetic acid.

Table 5.2 Patient education sheet

What is salicylic acid?

Salicylic acid in various preparations is commonly used in various formulations to treat a variety of skin disorders ranging from acne to dandruff to warts. Warts are caused when a virus infects cells in the skin. Salicylic acid helps to remove warts by destroying these virus-infected cells and allowing new healthy skin cells to replace them.

Remember that warts are not easy to treat. It often takes many daily treatments over weeks or even months to get rid of warts, and there is no guarantee that this method of treatment will work for you.

How to use your salicylic acid treatment

1. Any film from previous treatments must be peeled off
2. Excess dead skin over or surrounding the wart should be scraped away. This may be done by using sandpaper, an emery board or a nail file
3. Next, soak the area around the wart in warm water for several minutes, then pat the area dry
4. Using an applicator, carefully apply the salicylic acid product to the wart, avoiding all surrounding normal skin
5. You may cover the wart with occlusive tape, especially in high-pressure areas such as the ball of the foot or to prevent rubbing by clothing
6. Repeat this process every night until the wart clears or for 6 weeks. You may take 2- to 3-day 'holidays' from treatment if the discomfort is too great
7. Call your physician if the warts have not cleared in 6 weeks, if you have any problems with excessive pain or if you notice any signs that the wart is coming back

the area of the wart, left in place overnight and changed each day.[14] There is an alternative treatment for multiple flat warts, as described by Rees[3] who recommends 1% tannic acid and 2% salicylic acid in 40% alcohol or bay rum, rubbed into the wart areas twice a day.

There are more variations in the usage of MCAA, DCAA and TCAA. As with the use of salicylic acid, excess keratotic tissue should be trimmed before applying the acid solution. Strengths varying from 50% to 95% can be applied to the wart,[18,19] and must be done with an applicator once a week by the physician, who must be careful to avoid the surrounding healthy tissue. After application of this product, the wart and surrounding skin turn white. The application may be repeated weekly until resolution is seen, or for 4 weeks, or as long as continued improvement is noted.[8,19] Treatment at the surgery using these products is favored over podophyllin in pregnant patients.

ADVERSE EFFECTS (Table 5.3)

As these acids are used topically for treating warts, there are relatively few side effects. The most commonly reported side effects for salicylic acid are tenderness and local irritation of the treatment area, which usually resolve rapidly after treatment is discontinued.[8,14] A rare case of pyogenic granuloma after combined salicylic acid treatment and cryotherapy has been reported in the literature.[25] When flat warts on the face are treated with salicylic acid, there is a lower threshold for skipping treatment when inflammation is considerable to prevent post-inflammatory hyper- and hypopigmentation in this area. An extremely rare event in the case of topical administration to large numbers of warts over a broad surface area would be salicylic acid poisoning, which manifests itself by signs and symptoms of confusion, dizziness, headache, tachypnoea and tinnitus. Although package inserts warn

Table 5.3 Adverse effects of acids

Acid	Local effects	Systemic effects
Salycylic acid	Tenderness Local irritation Pyogenic granuloma (rare) Hypopigmentation and hyperpigmentation	Salicylic acid poisoning (extremely rare from topical use): confusion, dizziness, headache, tachypnoea, tinnitus
MCAA, BCAA, TCAA	Local discomfort Superficial ulceration Scab formation Excessive pain and soreness	

against use of salicylic acid in patients with diabetes, it is possible to use this modality under a physician's supervision, recognizing that there is an increased risk of infection and slower healing in these patients. Other patients with delayed wound healing or peripheral vascular disease should also visit the physician regularly to monitor therapy.

Similarly, most adverse effects reported with the use of MCAA, DCAA and TCAA are related to local effects of the acid, with the most commonly reported being local discomfort, superficial ulceration, scab formation, and excessive pain and soreness at the area of treatment.[7,9,17,18]

COST–BENEFIT CONSIDERATIONS

There are several advantages to the use of salicylic acid. As it is available over the counter, the patient does not require a prescription or even an appointment with a healthcare professional. The treatment is inexpensive; one formulation, Duofilm, costs about 33 cents per treatment.[22] It is also easily used and controlled by the patient and is relatively free

of significant side effects. Disadvantages of salicylic acid include its demand for daily involvement leading to the potential for poor compliance by the patient.[10,24]

Use of the other acids results in greater expense because usually the physician needs to apply this acid, e.g. TCAA is more expensive than most other options; the cost of achieving 100% clearance of simple condylomata is $US684, whereas extensive condylomata cost $US1288 with a mean of $US986.[19] Although these acids have side effects related mostly to local irritative effects, their expense, the need for administration by a physician and the availability of other well-reported options for physician-applied therapy have limited their use.

CASE REPORTS

Case 1

A 17-year-old high school football player presented with a 6-week history of a wart on the right ball of the foot. It had been sore when he ran, prompting his visit. The patient was having football practice every day and

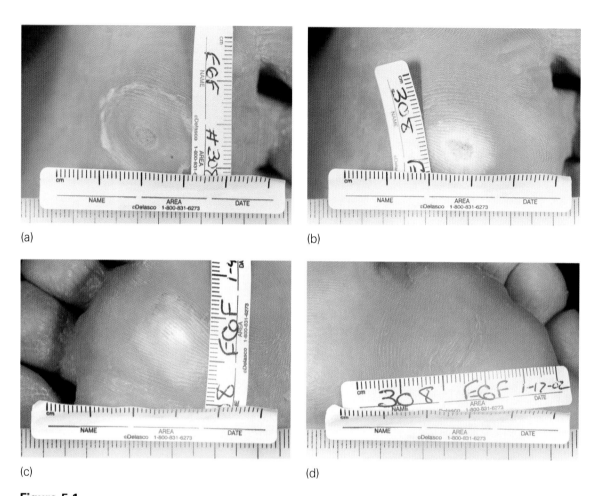

(a)   (b)

(c)   (d)

Figure 5.1

(a) A 7 × 8 mm diameter verrucous lesion with a few thrombosed capillaries is noted. Callusing is present on the surrounding skin. (b) The area of the wart now appears white after treatment with salicylic acid for 3 weeks. Thrombosed capillaries are still apparent. (c) At 8 weeks, the wart appears to be clear with some white discoloration of the skin remaining. The dermatoglyphs can be seen to move through the area where the wart was present in the past. (d) No evidence of the wart is present 2 months after discontinuation of therapy.

wanted to have a treatment that he could do at home which would not cause any pain or limit him from practising or playing football. Physical examination revealed a 7 × 8 mm diameter verrucous lesion with thrombosed capillaries and some slight callusing of the surrounding skin (Figure 5.1a). The patient was treated with 17% salicylic acid in a polyacrylic vehicle base once a day to the wart, filing it down each evening. After 3 weeks, the wart and surrounding skin had a white appearance and the wart was somewhat flatter (Figure 5.1b). The patient continued his treatment and 8 weeks after initiating therapy the wart

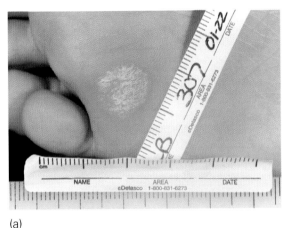
(a)

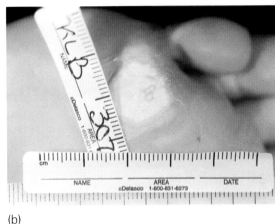
(b)

Figure 5.2
(a) A 1.4 × 1.2 cm diameter verrucous lesion with callusing is present on the right foot at the base of the fifth toe over the metatarsal head. (b) White discoloration typical of salicylic acid-treated warts, although the wart remains despite this treatment.

appeared to be gone (Figure 5.1c). Two months later, the patient visited the doctor for another problem and the wart was entirely clear (Figure 5.1d).

Case 2

A 18-year-old woman presented for evaluation of a wart on the right lateral foot at the base of the fifth toe over the metatarsal head. The patient was away at college and wanted to have a treatment that she could use while away and would not need physician follow-up. Physical examination revealed a 1.4 × 1.2 cm diameter verrucous lesion with slight brown coloration (Figure 5.2a). The patient treated the wart every day with salicylic acid in a polyacrylic vehicle base. She filed it each evening. Four weeks later she had noted very little improvement, and 8 weeks later the area

was white from denaturation of the proteins in the area with the salicylic acid although the wart persisted (Figure 5.2b). At this point the patient was home from college and the area was treated with liquid nitrogen cryotherapy every 2 weeks for three sessions; at that point the wart had cleared.

REFERENCES

1. Allen AL, Siegfried EC. What's new in human papillomavirus infection. *Curr Opin Pediatr* 2000; **12**: 365–9.
2. Chevalier, Andrew. *The Encyclopedia of Medicinal Plants*. New York: DK Publishing, 1996.
3. Rees RB. Warts. *Cutis* 1979; **23**: 588–93.
4. Van Brederode RL, Engel ED. Combined cryotherapy/70% salicylic acid treatment for plantar verrucae. *J Foot Ankle Surg* 2001; **40**: 36–41.

5. Huber C, Christophers E. Keratolytic effect of salicylic acid. *Arch Dermatol* 1977; **257**: 293–7.

6. Sterling JC, Handfield-Jones S, Hudson PM. Guidelines for the management of cutaneous warts. *Br J Dermatol* 2001; **144**: 4–11.

7. Gabriel G, Thin RN. Treatment of anogenital warts: comparison of trichloracetic acid and podophyllin versus podophyllin alone. *Br J Vener Dis* 1983; **59**: 124–6.

8. Goldfarb MT, Gupta AK, Gupta MA, Sawchuk WSD. Office therapy for human papillomavirus infection in nongenital sites. *Dermatol Clin* 1991; **9**: 287–6.

9. Steele K, Irwin WG. Treatment options for cutaneous warts in family practice. *J Fam Pract* 1988; **5**: 314–19.

10. Marchese Johnson S. Management of cutaneous warts: an evidence-based approach. *Cutis* 2002; in press.

11. Bunney MH. The treatment of plantar warts with 5-fluorouracil. *Br J Dermatol* 1973; **89**: 96.

12. Tidy G, Christie R, Whitefield M. Treating viral warts with a novel salicylic acid gel. *Practitioner* 1989; **233**: 467–8.

13. Bart BJ, Biglow J, Vance JC, Neveaux JL. Salicylic acid in karaya gum patch as a treatment for verruca vulgaris. *J Am Acad Dermatol* 1989; **20**: 74–6.

14. Bender ME, Schultz PP, Neveaux JL, Bush L. Nonmosaic verruca plantaris: treatment with a salicylic acid polymeric matrix delivery system. *Cutis* 1991; **47**: 199–200.

15. Parish LC, Monro E, Rex IH. Treatment of common warts with high-potency (26%) salicylic acid. *Clin Ther* 1988; **10**: 462–6.

16. NHS Research and Development: Center for Evidence Based Medicine. http://cebm. jr2.ox. ac.uk/

17. Godley MJ, Bradbeer CS, Gellan M, Thin RN. Cryotherapy compared with trichloroacetic acid in treating genital warts. *Genitourin Med* 1987; **63**: 390–2.

18. Abdullah AN, Walzman M, Wade A. Treatment of external genital warts comparing cryotherapy (liquid nitrogen) and trichloroacetic acid. *Sex Transm Dis* 1993; **20**: 344–5.

19. Alam M, Stiller M. Direct medical costs for surgical and medical treatment of condylomata accuminata. *Arch Dermatol* 2001; **137**: 337–41.

20. Dagnall JC. Monochloroacetic acid and verrucae. *Br J Chir* 1976; **41**: 105–7.

21. Dutta RK. Treatment of plantar warts by chemosurgery. A new technique. *Indian Med Gazette* 1983; **117**: 70.

22. Campbell BJ. The treatment of warts. *Prim Care* 1986; **13**: 465–76.

23. Bolton RA. Nongenital warts: classification and treatment options. *Am Fam Physician* 1991; **43**: 2049–56.

24. Miller DM, Brodell RT. Human papillomavirus infection: treatment options for warts. *Am Fam Physician* 1996; **53**: 135–43.

25. Kolbusz RV, O'Donoghue MN. Pyogenic granuloma following treatment of verruca vulgaris with cryotherapy and Duoplant. *Cutis* 1991; **47**: 204.

6 Imiquimod

Susannah Lambird Collier and Sandra Marchese Johnson

Historical aspects · Basic science · Clinical evidence · Favored treatment methodology · Adverse effects · Cost–benefit considerations · Course/prognosis · Case reports · References

HISTORICAL ASPECTS

Imiquimod (Aldara Cream, 3M Pharmaceuticals, St Paul, MN) is a topical immune response modifier that was approved by the Food and Drugs Administration (FDA) in 1997 for the treatment of external genital warts. Its development was inspired by successful studies with injectable interferon-α, a protein secreted by the body's innate defense system that enhances the destruction of virally infected cells. The goal was to create an immunomodulating drug that could be self-applied at home, thereby reducing costly, frequent, and potentially embarrassing surgery visits. Since its introduction, imiquimod has been used not only for anogenital warts, but also for verruca plana, molluscum contagiosum, herpes simplex, basal cell carcinomas, actinic keratoses, lentigo maligna, and acute tattoo removal. This chapter focuses on imiquimod and its role in home-based wart therapy.

BASIC SCIENCE

Imiquimod, also known as R-837 or S-26308, is an imidazoquinoline amine with the chemical name: 1-(2-methlypropyl)-1H-imidazo[4,5-c] quinolin-4-amine. The exact mechanism of action of imiquimod is not clearly understood; however, it appears to act through immune system modulation. The innate immune system eliminates pathogens with phagocytic cells, whereas the acquired immune system depends on the recognition of foreign antigens presented on major histocompatibility complexes (MHCs) by antigen-presenting cells.[1] Imiquimod stimulates both arms of this system through the induction of cytokines, including interferon-α (IFNα), interleukins 1, 6, 8, 10, and 12 (IL1, IL6, IL8, IL10 and IL12), tumor necrosis factor α (TNFα), granulocyte colony-stimulating factor (G-CSF) and granulocyte–macrophage colony-stimulating factor (GM-CSF).[1] In animal studies, increases in concentration of IFNα and TNFα are seen at application sites as soon as 1–4 hours after application.[2] The increases in IFNα and IL12 lead to an increased production of IFNγ, a major component of the cell-mediated immune response.[1] In a study analyzing the interrelationship of wart clearance, cytokines, and human papillomavirus (HPV) gene products, an increase in the levels of TNFα mRNA, IFNα mRNA, IFNβ mRNA, and IFNγ mRNA was directly correlated with wart reduction. At the same time, levels of HPV DNA decreased.[3] Finally, imiquimod has been proven to activate Langerhans' cells and enhance their migration to draining lymph nodes.[4] When applied topically, systemic absorption appears to be minimal. After a single topical application, less than 1% of the drug is recovered in the urine.[5]

CLINICAL EVIDENCE

Several randomized, double-blind, placebo-controlled studies have been using imiquimod on anogenital warts. In comparing 5% imiquimod cream with 1% imiquimod cream, the 5% strength has consistently shown better efficacy.[6,7] Based on intent-to-treat analyses, the percentage of patients with clearing of baseline warts using 5% compared with 1% imiquimod cream was 50% versus 21% in one study[6] (three times a week dosing) and 52% versus 14% in another study[7] (daily treatment).

To determine the optimal dosing regimen, comparisons were made of imiquimod applied three times a week, once daily, twice daily, and three times daily. This study concluded that dosing three times a week allowed for optimal clearance of genital warts while minimizing local adverse events.[8]

The percentage of patients with complete clearance of warts (using 5% imiquimod cream three times a week) appears to vary based on sex. In two predominantly male studies, complete clearance rates were 35%[10] and 27%. Another study, which had an even mix of male and female participants, analyzed the numbers based on sex. Complete clearance rates were 72% for females and 33% for males.[6] Several theories have been proposed to explain why women have better success with topical imiquimod. Some suspect that drug penetration may be greater through partially keratinized skin such as that of the vulva, as opposed to the fully keratinized skin on the penile shaft.[7] Others propose that there may be sex-specific differences in the amount or type of cytokines induced by imiquimod.[8]

Recurrence rates for patients whose warts had cleared varied from 13%[6] (three times a week application with a 12-week follow-up) to 19%[7] (daily application with a 10-week follow-up). Neither study detected a difference in recurrence rate based on sex. These rates are minimal when compared with many other modalities where recurrence rates are in the 50% range.

Very few studies have been done to investigate the use of imiquimod for common warts. One non-randomized, non-placebo-controlled, open-label study was done to evaluate the efficacy of 5% imiquimod cream applied five-times a week to verruca vulgaris resistant to previous treatment. Total clearance was achieved by 30% of patients after a mean treatment period of 9.2 weeks, and no recurrences of warts occurred in the treated area during a mean follow-up period of 32 weeks.[10] Based on their own clinical experience, some dermatologists have concluded that imiquimod is not effective when used as monotherapy for verruca vulgaris.[11] Using adjunctive therapy such as liquid nitrogen cryotherapy, or salicylic acid in the morning before imiquimod application, may be helpful. This may thin the wart, disrupt the stratum corneum, and allow the imiquimod to be better absorbed, enhancing its effectiveness. Double-blind placebo-controlled studies are needed to evaluate this approach.

As for verruca planae, few clinical studies have been done to evaluate the efficacy of imiquimod. One recent case report demonstrated clerance of multiple, treatment-resistant verrucae planae on the dorsal hands of a 42-year-old man after 6 weeks of treatment three times a week using 5% imiquimod cream.[12]

The strength of the evidence supporting the use of imiquimod in the treatment of genital and perianal warts can be estimated using the scale of the Oxford Centre for Evidence Based Medicine. As there are multiple randomized controlled studies with homogeneity of results, the treatment of genital warts is supported by level 1 evidence (see Chapter 19).

Using the same criteria to determine the use of imiquimod for non-genital warts, the recommendations would be a rating of IV. This recommendation is based only on case studies and not on randomized controlled studies (see Chapter 19).

FAVORED TREATMENT METHODOLOGY (Table 6.1)

For anogenital warts, imiquimod should be applied in a thin layer, directly to the warts, three times a week at bedtime. It should remain, unoccluded, on the skin for 6–10 hours and must then be washed off with mild soap and water. Treatment should continue until there is a total clearance of anogenital warts, or for a maximum of 16 weeks. A rest period of several days may be taken in the case of an uncomfortable local skin reaction.[14] Because this medication is expensive, when an entire packet is not required for a single treatment, we save the open packet, seal it in a zip-lock bag and refrigerate it, so long as the remaining medication is used within 1 week. This approach is not recommended by the manufacturer because it has not been scientifically tested.

For resistant common warts, we use imiquimod cream three times a week in the evening as an adjunct to various destructive therapies. We also use destructive home therapies to improve the efficacy of imiquimod.

Table 6.1 Favored treatment methodology

1. Wash the involved area with soap and water, then dry
2. A thin coating of 5% imiquimod cream is applied three times week at bedtime
3. Wash off with mild soap and water 6–10 hours later
4. Continue until warts are gone, for a maximum of 16 weeks

Each morning, salicylic acid is applied topically and each evening the warts are filed with an emery board, soaked in water for 5 minutes and then patted dry, before application of imiquimod three times a week.

ADVERSE EFFECTS

Adverse reactions to topical 5% imiquimod are generally mild and limited to local irritation. In one large, multicenter trial, the most common reactions were erythema (67%), erosions (32.1%), excoriation or flaking (24.5%), edema (16%), scabbing (15.1%), and induration (8.5%). Most reactions were mild. Moderate erythema was present in 34% of patients whereas 5.7% had the severe form; 10.4% and 0.9% of the two groups, respectively, experienced moderate-to-severe erosions, and 5.7% and 0.9% had moderate-to-severe excoriation or flaking. All other moderate-to-severe reactions were experienced by less than 5% of patients.[6]

In one study, 6 weeks after discontinuation of the trial, a patient experienced a stricturing of the penile foreskin caused by local skin irritation which necessitated circumcision. This was partially attributed to imiquimod application and partially to the warts. For this reason, it is advised that uncircumcised men who apply imiquimod under the foreskin should be instructed to retract the foreskin daily and wash and dry the area thoroughly.[13]

COST–BENEFIT CONSIDERATIONS

Aldara is supplied in single-use packets, each containing 250 mg of the cream (12.5 mg imiquimod), sufficient to cover a wart area of up to 20 cm^2.[14] The average wholesale price of a 12-packet box is $US124.80.[14]

A recent analysis[13] was done comparing the costs of different modalities used to treat

Table 6.2 Patient education sheet

What is imiquimod?

Imiquimod is a protein that stimulates your body to defend itself against the wart virus. Warts are difficult to treat and there is no guarantee that this method of treatment will work for you

Before treatment

Wash and dry the affected areas using mild soap and water

During treatment

Imiquimod is to be applied in a thin layer, directly to the warts, three times a week at bedtime. After 6–10 hours, it must be washed off with mild soap and water. If you are an uncircumcised man, washing should be done a minimum of twice a day, taking special care to retract the foreskin completely. Treatment should continue until there is total clearance of the warts, or for a maximum of 16 weeks. A rest period of several days is permitted if an uncomfortable local skin reaction occurs

After treatment

Call your physician if you have a fever or if the local skin reactions do not improve within a day or two

condylomata acuminata. Although the authors did not take into consideration long-term efficacy, recurrence rates, and patient preferences, they were able to draw some useful conclusions. On average, surgical modalities, including excision, electrodesiccation, LEEP, and laser treatment, were less expensive than medical treatments. Of course, these surgical treatments can lead to significant scarring and often require a highly trained operator using costly equipment. Imiquimod was calculated, on average, to be the third most expensive medical modality, behind both interferon-α_{2b} and podophyllum resin. As with podofilox, the advantage of imiquimod is the ability of patients to self-apply the medication. This reduces the need for multiple, costly visits to the doctor's office, and allows patients to treat themselves in the privacy of their own homes. Of the two patient-applied therapies, imiquimod was approximately three times as expensive as podofilox ($US1255 per complete clearance of the average condyloma vs $US424). The difference in cost was the result of the expense of the medication. If the recurrence rate is less with imiquimod cream compared with podofilox, as it would appear from analysis of current evidence, the costs of permanent clearing of warts would converge.

COURSE/PROGNOSIS

Imiquimod, used three times a week, seems to be an effective yet costly alternative to treating condylomata accuminata (Table 6.2). The ideal use for this medication would be for a woman with genital warts on the vulva or as an adjunctive treatment in a patient with warts resistant to other therapies. The course can be long, up to 16 weeks in patients treated with monotherapy, but side effects are minimal and clearance rates approach 75%. Men with condylomata on the shaft of the penis, on the other hand, should be forewarned that the success rate is much lower. In fact only about one-third will have complete resolution of their genital warts. If cleared, both sexes have an equal chance of recurrence, about 15%.

CASE REPORTS

Case 1

A 23-year-old white man presented with 75 0.1–2.0 mm warts on the shaft of his penis. A

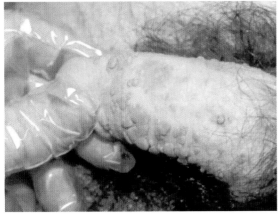

(a)

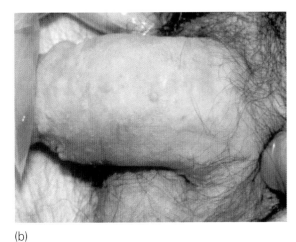

(b)

Figure 6.1
(a) A patient presented with scores of 0.1–2 mm diameter warts on the shaft of his penis. (b) Four weeks after monotherapy with 5% imiquimod cream three times a week, fewer than a dozen warts remained. These warts subsequently cleared over the next 3 weeks.

few similar warts were present in the pubic area and the groin (Figure 6.1a). These warts had first appeared 18 months earlier; there had been no previous treatment. The 5% imiquimod cream was applied three times a

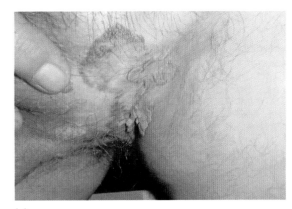

(a)

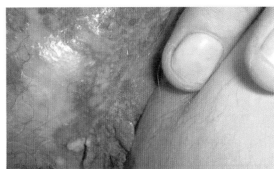

(b)

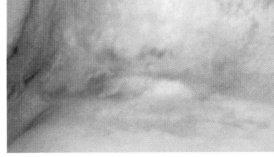

(c)

Figure 6.2
(a) A 5 × 4-cm condyloma is present in the left inguinal fold. (b) The wart is greatly improved 6 weeks later after using 5% imiquimod cream three times a week as monotherapy. (c) The wart is almost clear at 10 weeks with continued imiquimod cream three times a week as monotherapy.

week at bedtime. He developed mild erythema and irritation, but was able to maintain his treatment schedule. Four weeks later only nine warts remained (Figure 6.1b). Seven weeks later he was completely clear. There have been no recurrences.

Case 2

A 26-year-old woman presented with a 5 × 4 cm condyloma in the left inguinal fold (Figure 6.2a). After consideration of the risks and benefits, 5% imiquimod cream was applied five times a week at bedtime to the wart. Erythema, tenderness, and edema were noted in the treated area but the patient was able to maintain the same treatment schedule throughout the course of therapy. Six weeks later the wart was greatly improved (Figures 6.2b). With continued treatment the wart has resolved at 10 weeks (Figure 6.2c). By 12 weeks the wart was entirely clear and there were no recurrent lesions at a follow-up visit 1 year later.

REFERENCES

1. Sauder DN. Immunomodulatory and pharmacologic properties of imiquimod. *J Am Acad Dermatol* 2000; **43S**: S6–11.
2. Imbertson LM, Beaurline JM, Couture AM et al. Cytokine induction in hairless mouse and rat skin after topical application of the immune response modifiers imiquimod and S-28463. *J Invest Dermatol* 1998; **110**: 734–9.
3. Tyring SK, Arany I, Stanley MA et al. A randomized, controlled, molecular study of condylomata acuminata clearance during treatment with imiquimod. *J Infect Dis* 1998; **178**: 551–5.
4. Suzuki H, Wang B, Shivji GM et al. Imiquimod, a topical immune response modifier, induces migration of Langerhans cells. *J Invest Dermatol* 2000; **114**: 135–41.
5. Slade HB, Owens ML, Tomai MA, Miller RL. Imiquimod 5% cream (Aldara). *Exp Opin Invest Drugs* 1998; **7**: 437–49.
6. Edwards L, Ferenczy A, Eron L et al. Self-administered topical 5% imiquimod cream for external anogenital warts. *Arch Dermatol* 1998; **134**: 25–30.
7. Beutner KR, Tyring SK, Trofatter SF et al. Imiquimod, a patient-applied immune-response modifier for treatment of external genital warts. *Antimicrob Agents Chemother* 1998; **42**: 789–94.
8. Fife KH, Ferenczy A, Douglas JM et al. *Sex Transm Dis* 2001; **28**: 226–31.
9. Beutner KR, Spruance SL, Hougham AJ et al. Treatment of genital warts with an immune-response modifier (imiquimod). *J Am Acad Dermatol* 1998; **38**: 230–9.
10. Hengge UR, Esser S, Schultewolter R et al. Self-administered topical 5% imiquimod for the treatment of common warts and molluscum contagiosum. *Br J Dermatol* 2000; **143**: 1026–31.
11. Proceedings of a Clinical Roundtable. Immune response modifier therapy: Treatment of warts, basal cell carcinoma and actinic keratosis. *Skin and Allergy News* 2001; **10**(suppl).
12. Oster-Schmidt C. Imiquimod: A new possibility for treatment-resistant verrucae planae. *Arch Dermatol* 2001; **137**: 666–7.
13. 3M Pharmaceuticals. *Aldara (Imiquimod) Cream. 5% Product Monograph.* 7 St Paul, MN: 3M Pharmaceuticals, 1997.
14. Alam M, Stiller M. Direct medical costs for surgical and medical treatment of condylomata acuminata. *Arch Dermatol* 2001; **157**: 337–41.

7 Podophyllin

Pradip Bhattacharjee and Robert T Brodell

Historical aspects • Basic science • Clinical evidence • Favored treatment methodology • Adverse effects • Cost–benefit considerations • Case reports • References

Podophyllins are a crude extract of cytotoxic chemicals obtained from the common plant *Podophyllum peltatum* (mandrake or May apple) and *Podophyllum emodi*. It is a lipid-soluble compound that causes tissue necrosis and is commonly used in the treatment of genital warts. The exact mechanism of action is uncertain. It is known to arrest cell division, and cause cell death.[1] Podofilox, also called podophyllotoxin (Condylox), is a purer, more active, and stable form of podophyllin. Podophyllins have been widely used for condyloma treatment since the 1940s.[2] Currently, the drug is routinely used as both a patient-administered home treatment and a physician-applied treatment in the surgery.

HISTORICAL ASPECTS

The use of podophyllins dates back to pre-colonial times in the USA. It was used by Native American tribes as a purgative and an effective antidote for snake bites.[3] The resin of the dried May apple rhizomes and roots was prepared by boiling it in alcohol. The alcohol evaporated until the substance turned syrupy. Cold water was added and the mixture was allowed to stand for 24 hours to precipitate the resin.[4] The precipitate was collected by strain-ing and the product was dried at 80°F (27°C). Its approximate yield was 84 pounds of resin per ton of root. It is not known whether the Native Americans first discovered the use of mandrake by trial and error or accidentally.[5,6] Many tribes also used the formula to treat intestinal worms. The Penobscot tribes were the first to use May apple for external use in the treatment of warts on the skin. The Huron and Iroquois tribes used the plant as an anti-rheumatic, cathartic, dermatological aid, ear medicine, insecticide, and laxative. Other Cherokee tribes were described using the root as a purgative, vermifuge, and anti-helminthic. Native Americans introduced the plant to the settlers of the New World. In the colonies the root was used as a topical antidote for snake bites. Additionally, it was used to stimulate 'glands' in the treatment of gastrointestinal disorders and rheumatism.

Even during the 1800s, the thin rhizome and root of the plant *Podophyllum peltatum* was recognized to be the most poisonous part.[5] It was ironically also noted to be the most useful part. Since the 1820s the plant has been recognized as being of medicinal value in the official US Pharmacopeia.

It was not until 1942 that interest in podophyllin was renewed as a topical treatment for condyloma accuminatum.[2] Kaplan applied the compound to various warts and found it to be very effective in both genital and non-genital locations.

It was shown, during the 1970s, that the resin of both *Podophyllum peltatum* and *emodi* contained many biologically active compounds that had anti-mitotic actions, which resulted in keratolysis and subsequent eradication of warts.[7] As a result of the drug's potency, it was the standard of care for physicians to administer the drug in the surgery. After many studies in the laboratory, it was shown that podofilox (podophyllotoxin) was the most active ingredient of podophyllin.[8–11]

The discovery that podophyllins inhibited cell mitosis led to its study for the treatment of basal cell carcinoma.[12] Initial trials showed a high relapse rate and the use of the drug for experimentation was discontinued. Subsequently, two semi-synthetic derivatives of podophyllin, etoposide and teniposide, were developed which have shown therapeutic activity in many neoplasms.

BASIC SCIENCE

Podophyllin is a resin mixture obtained from dried rhizomes and roots of the ubiquitous plants *Podophyllin emodi* and *Podophyllin peltatum* (May apple or mandrake), which are grown in the Himalayas and North America, respectively.[12] *Podophyllum peltatum* is a perennial native herb found growing in moist soils in wooded and pastoral regions of eastern North America.[6] These plants are found in the eastern regions from southern Maine to Florida and west to Texas and Minnesota. The plant gets its generic name from the Greek words *pous* and *phyllon*, meaning foot-shaped leaves. The plant grows to about 18 inches (46 cm) high, with dark-green multilobed leaves resembling an umbrella – hence it is sometimes called 'umbrella plant'. The leaves protect the large white flower growing between them. The plant flowers from March

to May, and fruits ripen from May to August. The roots of the plant are dark-brown, fibrous, and jointed. The leaves and roots were found to be extremely poisonous; however, resin mixtures obtained from the rhizome and roots yield the chemical podophyllin.

Podophyllin resin is an amorphous powder, light brown to yellow in color, which turns darker when subjected to light.[12] It is a mixture of ligands, with podophyllotoxin (podofilox) being the major component. Smaller concentrations of α- and β-peltatins, picrophodophyllotoxins and demethylpodophyllotoxins are also found within the resin.[14] There is variation in the proportion of these ligands depending on the specific batch and species of podophyllums.

Podofilox (Condylox (Condylox™, *Dak Pharmaceuticals, Philadelphia, PA, USA*)) a major active component of podophyllin, has a molecular weight of 414.4 daltons.[15] It is sparingly soluble in water and completely soluble in alcohols. Its chemical name is [5*R*-(5α,5aβ,8aα,9α]-5,8,8a,9-tetrahydro-9-hydroxy-5-(3,4,5-trimethoxyphenyl)furo[3′,4′:6,7]naphtho-[2,3,-*d*]-1,3-dioxol-6(5a*H*)-one. The structure of podofilox (Figure 7.1) has five rings.

In 1942, Kaplan[2] introduced the use of topical podophyllin in the management and treatment of warts. Initially, Kaplan thought the

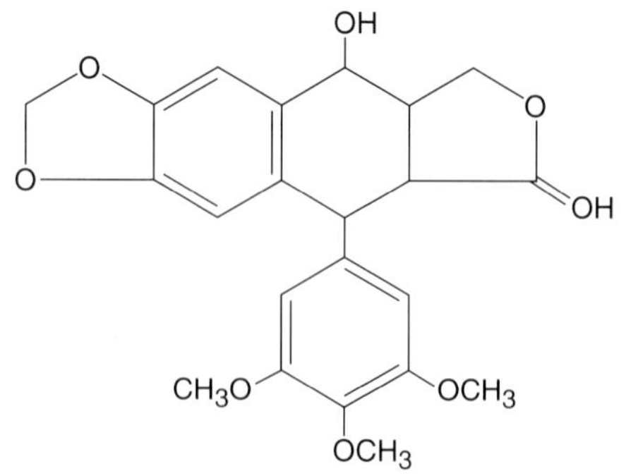

Figure 7.1
Molecular structure of podofilox.

mechanism of action was to induce potent vasospasm, with subsequent ischemia, necrosis, and eventual sloughing. Kaplan realized that this theory could not be confirmed by histologic methods. Many other scientists believed that podophyllin had a direct toxic effect on the human papillomavirus. Clinical trials subsequently showed that the resin of podophyllin simulated the action of the anti-gout drug colchicine.[2] It worked by arresting cell division (mitosis) in metaphase, which subsequently caused epithelial cell death.

The inhibition of mitosis caused by podophyllin was attributed to the drug's ability to interact with and inhibit the mitotic spindle.[16] The drug adheres to the cell proteins and increases amino acid incorporation. Its actions also include inhibition of the synthesis of purine and incorporation into RNA. The drug can, in addition, reduce the activity of cytochrome oxidase and succinoxidase within the mitochondria.[14]

In 1984 Wade and Ackerman[17] studied the histological changes of condyloma acuminatum after the application of podophyllin resin. They found pallor of the epidermis, secondary to intracellular and intercellular edema, and necrosis in the lower half of the epidermis with numerous mitoses. Lymphocytic, histiocytic, and neutrophilic infiltrates are present within the papillary dermis. The most intense changes occur within the first 48 hours of treatment. The changes of podophyllin treatment can be differentiated from squamous cell carcinoma by the maturation of the keratinocytes and absence of dyskeratosis. By 72 hours after treatment, the necrotic keratinocytes are seen in the upper epidermis with few mitoses. After 1 week, the histologic changes are absent.

CLINICAL EVIDENCE

As mentioned earlier, in 1941 Kaplan rejuvenated interest and first published an article about the use of podophyllin resin in the treatment of warts.[2] He used a single application of 25% podophyllin admixed in mineral oil and applied it directly to the 'condylomatous masses'. The patient began to feel pain over the area after 6–8 hours. After 12 hours, there was local inflammation and edema at the site of application. There was sloughing of the tissue with resolution of pain after 2–3 days. The area of application returned to normal without scarring on days 4–5. Kaplan also studied 20 patients with condylomata acuminata and found that all the patients were cured. Kaplan cited a few specific cases with no recurrences but did not specifically address the exact recurrence rate in this study.

In 1948 Sullivan et al. confirmed the efficacy of the active ingredient of podophyllin, podophyllotoxin (podofilox), in the treatment of condylomata acuminata.[13] They treated 44 patients with condylomata acuminata with alcoholic solutions of non-crystalline podophyllotoxin. The results showed an 81.5% cure rate with a variable number of applications ranging from one to five. This study showed similar efficacy rates to those of Kaplan without addressing the recurrence rates.

In 1976 Vaughan et al.[18] described in detail the histological changes associated with podophyllin therapy on genital warts. The microscopic findings included acanthosis, numerous mitoses, vacuolated epidermal cells, and chronic inflammation. Other microscopic changes included disappearance of melanin in the basal layer at the region of application.

The clinical evidence supporting the use of podophyllin as a treatment for genital warts is presented in Table 7.1. The percentage of patients cleared with administration of podophyllin was between 22% and 100%, and the recurrence rate varied from 0% to 79%, with most cases having recurrence rates of less than 25%. There are several major differences in the methodology of these studies highlighted in Table 7.1. Specifically, the concentration and type of podophyllin utilized

Table 7.1 Clinical studies using podophyllin therapy

Author	Type of study	No. of patients	Percentage cleared	Recurrence rate (%)	Special notes
Kaplan[2]	Cohort	20	80	N/R	Podophyllin resin applied directly to area to treat genital warts. Used 20% podophyllin solution
Sullivan et al[13]	Cohort	35	80	N/R	Application with 20% podophyllin solution
Vaughan et al[18]	Animal research	1	N/A	N/R	Treated a 5-year-old thoroughbred chestnut mare with multiple lesions over vulva and perianal area. Topical applications of 20% podophyllin in 95% ethyl alcohol produced rapid involution
Bunney et al[19]	Meta-analysis	1802	81	N/R	Studied series of 11 comparative wart treatment trials undertaken between 1969 and 1975. Assessment after 12 weeks of treatment
Von Krogh[20]	Randomized comparative study	227	43	13	Compared alcoholic solutions with 20% podophyllin, 8% podophyllotoxin and 8% colchicine; showed similar clearance; 43% permanently cleared taking into account the recurrence rate
Simmons[21]	Randomized, comparative double-masked study	109 males	22 (without recurrence)	0	Compared 10% and 25% podophyllin in tincture of benzoin compound; 22% free of warts
Von Krogh[9]	Randomized, comparative double-masked study	214 men	54, 48	N/R	54% clearance in 41 men treated in office with 8% podophyllotoxin in ethanol; 48% clearance in 173 men who self-administered topical preparation of 0.5–1% podophyllotoxin
Bashi[22]	Cohort	206	51	N/R	Patients treated with podophyllin required a mean of 6.7±SD 3.5 treatments over a mean of 4.7±SD 2.4 weeks.
Jensen[23]	Cohort	30	76.6	43%(at 3 months)	Recurrence rates: 43% at 3 months, 56% at 6 months, 56% at 9 months, 65% at 12 months

Table 7.1 continued

Author	Type of study	No. of patients	Percentage cleared	Recurrence rate (%)	Special notes
Lim et al[24]	Randomized, comparative clinical trial	64 men	66, 72	N/R	Used 25% podophyllin application 66% clearance in patients with hospital application 72% clearance in patients with self-application
Von Krogh[25]	Cohort	61	70, 63	N/R	Used 0.5% podophyllotoxin in ethanol applied twice daily 70% clearance with 4-day trial 63% clearance with 5-day trial.
Lassus[26]	Randomized, comparative clinical trial	100 men	100 (0.5% podophyllo-toxin), 71 (20% podophyllin)	23 (0.5% podophyllo-toxin), 38 (20% podophyllin)	Compared 0.5% podophyllotoxin and 20% podophyllin Clearance measured with one to four treatment cycles
Huwyler et al[27]	Comparative clinical trial	25	84.5 (30-day trial)	N/R	Used 0.5% solution of podophyllotoxin (condyline)
Beutner et al[11]	Comparative, double-masked clinical trial	56	73.6	N/R	Comparison of 0.5% podofilox and placebo treatments 73.6% clearance in podofilox vs 8.3% clearance in placebo-treated group.
Stone et al[28]	Randomized clinical trial	450	41	25	Podophyllin treatment showed 41% clearance using 6-weekly treatments 3 month clearance of 17% for podophyllin group
Kirby et al[29]	Double-masked, randomized clinical trial	38 men	53.3	79 after 2 weeks	0.5% podofilox treatment twice daily for 3 days a week for 4 weeks
Baker et al[30]	Comparative clinical trial	37 women	50	22	0.5% podofilox treatment twice daily for 3 days followed by 4 drug-free days Two to four treatment cycles given
Greenberg et al[31]	Double-masked, placebo-controlled study	72 women	74	N/R	Patient-applied 0.5% podofilox was compared with placebo group Application 3 days followed by 4 days without treatment 2- to 4-week cycles 74% clearance of podofilox and 18% clearance of placebo group

Table 7.1 continued

Author	Type of study	No. of patients	Percentage cleared	Recurrence rate (%)	Special notes
Von Krogh and Hellberg[32]	Double-masked, placebo-controlled study	60 women	43%, 66% 91% (after 1,2 and 3 treatment cycle)	14	Used 0.5% podophyllotoxin cream Applied twice daily in 3-day cycles once weekly for up to 3 weeks Complete and permanent cure in 38 of 44 patients (77%)
Syed and Lundin[33]	Comparative open study	60 men	100,100 and 70 (4-week cycle using 0.3% solution, 0.3% cream and 0.15% cream)	5.6 (after 16 weeks)	Compared clinical efficacy of 0.3% podophyllotoxin in both 70% ethanolic solution and cream preparation on genital warts Evaluated in 4-week cycles
Syed et al[34]	Placebo-controlled, double-masked study	80	68.3 (41/60 patients) 83 (349/420 warts)	10 (after 16 weeks)	Compared clinical efficacy and tolerance of 0.3% and 0.5 podophyllotoxin in cream emulsion
Von Krogh et al[35]	Placebo-controlled comparative study	57 men	72, 81 (treated with 0.25% or 0.5% podo-phyllotoxin)	38	Compared efficacy of 0.5% and 0.25% podophyllotoxin preparations in untreated penile wart 1–2 self-treatment twice daily for 3 days
Bonnez et al[36]	Double-masked, randomized, placebo-controlled study	103	68	19	Used 0.5% podofilox patient administration of anogenital warts
Aynaud and Tranbaloc[37]	Cohort	20	81 (balano-preputial and vulvar mucous membranes) 67 (keratinized tissue) 63 (anal margin)	16 (in mucous membranes)	Efficacy of podophylotoxin (0.5%) was assessed in the balanopreputial, vulvar, keratinized tissues and the anal margins
Hellberg et al[38]	Randomized clinical study	60 women	82 (podo-phyllotoxin) 59 (podophyllin solution)		Compared weekly application of 20% podophyllin solution or self-treatment with 0.5% podophyllotoxin cream twice daily for 3 days at weekly intervals

Table 7.1 continued

Author	Type of study	No. of patients	Percentage cleared	Recurrence rate (%)	Special notes
Strand et al[39]	Randomized controlled clinical study	90 men	44, 68, 74 and 78 (after 1, 2, 3 and) 4 cycles		Compared self-treatment of 0.15% cream, 0.3% cream and 0.5% solution of podophylotoxin Treatment twice daily for 3 days for four treatment cycles.
Petersen et al[40]	Randomized controlled, clinical trial	136	63	N/R	Comparison of topical podophyllotoxin cream 0.5% and podophyllotoxin solution 0.5% in genital warts Total of 136 and 133 wart lesions were treated with each preparation applied twice daily for 3 days, repeated with a 4-day interval for 2- to 4-week cycles
Claesson et al[41]	Controlled randomized prospective study	120	Males: 75.1, 79, 85.6 (in 0.15% cream, 0.3% cream, 0.5% solution) Females: 86.2, 92.6, 93.1 (for above preparations, respectively)	6 (0.15% cream), 8.6 (0.3% cream), 8.6 (0.5% solution)	Studied the efficacy and safety of two cream formulations of podophyllotoxin (0.15% and 0.3%) and 0.5% podophyllotoxin solution
Tyring et al[42]	Double-masked, randomized, multicenter, vehicle-controlled investigation	326	37.1 (0.5% podofilox gel) 2.3 (vehicle gel) with complete resolution	N/R	Comparison of 0.5% podofilox gel and vehicle gel after 4 weeks of therapy.
Longstaff and von Krogh[43]	Review of literature	N/A	N/A	N/A	Advocated the use of 0.15–0.5% purified podophyllotoxin preparations applied twice daily for 3 days
von Krogh and Longstaff[44]	Review of literature	N/A	N/A	N/A	Advocated the use of home treatment with podophyllotoxin as the first-line therapy for anogenital warts Advocated against the use of podophyllin because of its low efficacy, high toxicity

N/A, not applicable; N/R, not reported.

and their vehicles are critical differences. Other differences include the frequency of treatment, patient-applied treatment versus surgery/physician-instituted therapy, and the length of therapy. The stronger the concentration of the podophyllin, the better the response rate. Several types of podophyllin used show different clearance and recurrence rates. Podofilox has many advantages over podophyllin, including standard formulation and ease of patient-applied administration.[1] Podofilox has a decreased risk of systemic absorption compared with podophyllin.[11] It has also been reported[1] that podofilox is 'more effective' and shows 'faster resolution' of genital warts compared with podophyllin. The greater number of applications lead to greater resolution of the wart. The vehicle used for applying podophyllin was not as important as the concentration of the agent. It was generally shown in the literature that patient-applied treatments resulted in greater compliance over physician-applied podophyllin treatment.[1]

We can conclude from the evidence given that podophyllin and podophyllotoxin are very safe and effective modes of treatment for genital warts. It is advocated by many researchers in the field that it should be the first-line treatment of genital warts. Although there are contraindications (pregnancy, bronchial asthma, drug interactions, etc.), when used with careful clinical follow-up only a few modes of therapy (cryosurgery, simple surgical excision) can compare with its safety and efficacy. Using our modified Evidence-based Medicine scale, both podophyllin and podophyllotoxin are level 1 for the treatment of genital warts (see Chapter 19).

FAVORED TREATMENT METHODOLOGY

The favored treatment methodology varies according to whether the podophyllin is physi-

cian applied or patient applied. Patient-applied Condylox gel or solution has gained popularity over recent years.

We favor the use of Condylox gel with the following technique:[15] Condylox gel should be applied twice daily morning and evening (every 12 hours), for 3 consecutive days. The patient should then withhold use for 4 consecutive days. This 1-week cycle of treatment should be repeated for up to 4 weeks until the wart tissue disappears.

Condylox gel 0.5% or Condylox solution 0.5% should be applied to the wart with the cotton-tipped applicator coated with the drug.[15] Application on the normal area around the wart should be minimized. It is recommended that application should cover an area of 10 cm^2 or less of the wart tissue. No more than 0.5 ml of the gel should be used per day. The gel should be allowed to dry before there is any contact with other regions of the body. Patients should wash their hands thoroughly before and after each application of the gel, and dispose of the applicator after each use.

ADVERSE EFFECTS

Adverse effects of these drugs are generally mild and include local reactions at the application site.[15] The main adverse effects of topical podofilox are inflammation, burning, erosion, pain, itching, and bleeding. Less frequently reported complications include stinging, erythema, desquamation, scabbing, discoloration, tenderness, dryness, crusting, fissure, soreness, ulceration, swelling/edema, tingling, rash, and blisters. Rarely, systemic reactions occur, especially if the medication is administered for a longer period of time than recommended, used over a broad area, or ingested. Severe reactions usually occur within the first 2 weeks of treatment.

The most common systemic adverse effect of the drug was headaches.[15] Investigational studies using this drug systemically for cancer treatment show adverse systemic effects that include nausea, vomiting, fever, diarrhea, bone marrow suppression, and oral ulcerations. Other systemic toxicities using podophyllin resin included nausea, vomiting, fever, diarrhea, peripheral neuropathy, altered mental status, lethargy, coma, tachypnea, respiratory failure, leukocytosis, pancytosis, hematuria, renal failure, and seizures. Management of toxicities or adverse effects resulting from the application of topical medications should include thorough washing of the area of application and supportive care.

COST–BENEFIT CONSIDERATIONS

Two published articles have elucidated the cost-effectiveness of treatment of genital warts with podofilox therapy.[45,46] A study published by Monhanty in 1995 detailed the cost-effectiveness of 25% podophyllin resin and 0.5% podofilox solution in the treatment of genital warts.[47] The article showed that the average treatment cost for a course of podofilox was more than that for podophyllin resin (£20.75 versus £14.95, respectively). The cure rate was 66% in the group treated with podofilox and only 34.6% in the group treated with podophyllin. When the cost of secondary treatment options was compared between the two study groups, the cost per patient cured of warts with podophyllin resin was £27.15 compared with £25.73 for podofilox solution. There was no cost–benefit from use of physician-administered podophyllin resin, compared with patient-applied podofilox solution, although the latter was superior in its overall cure rate.

The second study, by Langley et al in 1999, was about the cost-effectiveness of two patient-applied versus provider-administered intervention strategies for the treatment of external genital warts.[46] The results showed that estimated costs for patients initially treated with podofilox gel was $US1304 and with imiquimod $US1265. They concluded that initial treatment with imiquimod is the preferred intervention option, because it yielded a 39% greater clearance rate than podofilox gel, while being 3% less costly. This reinforces the fact that a multitude of therapeutic modalities is available to treat patients with warts, and knowledge about the cost–benefit factors should be explained to the patient.

CASE REPORTS

Case 1

A 6-month-old baby girl presented for evaluation of 'skin tags' in the perianal area. There was no history of genital warts in the family, but the mother had warts on her hands. A thorough investigation by a local government agency charged with this task revealed no evidence of sexual abuse. Physical examination revealed a dozen papules of diameter 0.5–3 mm with verrucous surface features in the perianal area (Figure 7.2a). No warts were present elsewhere. The patient was treated with applications of 25% podophyllin in benzoin at the surgery. This was carefully applied with a Q-tip (Figure 7.2b). Ten days after the first treatment, the perianal skin showed white scaling and maceration (Figure 7.2c). The warts were considerably smaller but persisted. Podphyllin was applied to the remaining warts on two additional occasions, at which time the warts were completely clear. There was no recurrence over the next year.

Case 2

A 2-year-old boy presented with multiple perianal warts. There was no history of child

Table 7.2 Patient education sheet

What are podophyllins?

Podophyllins are a group of lipid-soluble, anti-mitotic compounds that cause tissue death (necrosis) and keratolysis; they are commonly used in the treatment of genital warts. The necrosis causes subsequent sloughing of tissue which destroys the wart physically. The main advantage of this particular treatment modality is that it does not involve cutting, which would leave scars, and there is a minimal amount of pain. It is important to understand that a single treatment may not cure the wart; multiple treatments may be required. The treatment approaches a 100% cure rate depending on which formula is used. There is no guarantee that this topical pharmacologic treatment will work for you. Other methods may be used if this one proves unsuccessful.

1. **Prior to treatment**
   The wart and the surrounding area are evaluated
   The physician will examine your wart
   The area of the wart is cleaned with alcohol prep
2. **During treatment**
   The doctor will apply the medicine to the warts during the surgery visit
   You will have a cold sensation as the solution is applied with a wooden applicator or cotton swab
   After the solution is dry, a gauze may be placed over the treatment site, depending on the location
   Tell your doctor about any side effects from the medication at the local site or other generalized symptoms
3. **After treatment**
   At the end of the 4-hour period, remove the gauze and wash the medicine off with soap and water
   Later in the day, you will notice that you have redness, scaly surface, or pain
   Call the physician if you have any problems with pain or other discomfort
   May need to come back to the physician's surgery for the wound to be débrided weekly
   Do not be upset if the warts do not disappear completely after a single administration. As we never know how deep a wart is, multiple applications may be required, especially if the wart is located in the palms and soles. Bleeding into the blister may occur, giving it a black color
   Warts may recur or a ring may remain after treatment. Please call our physician with any signs of recurrence

abuse or genital warts in the family. Physical examination revealed multiple perianal warts of diameter 1–4 mm (Figure 7.3a), with a verrucous surface. No warts were present elsewhere. The patient was treated with application of 25% podophyllin in benzoin at the surgery. This was applied with a Q-tip on to the perianal surface (Figure 7.3b). Subsequently, there was excellent improvement and after 7 days, a few tiny warts remained in a few areas (Figure 7.3c). A second treatment was applied (Figure 7.3d). One week after the second treatment, the warts appeared flatter. The patient remained clear when seen 4 weeks later (Figure 7.3e).

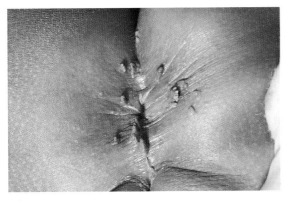

(a)

Figure 7.2
(a) Multiple perianal warts of diameter 0.5–3 mm present in the perianal region of a 6-month-old child. (b) The appearance of the perianal region immediately after application of 25% podophyllin in benzoin. (c) Macerated skin with focal 1-mm foci of residual wart 10 days after treatment. Additional treatment is required.

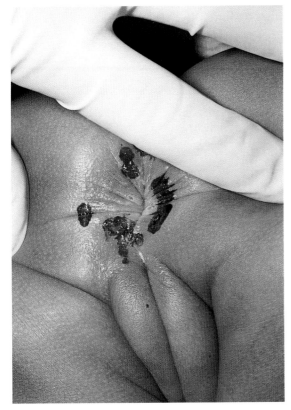

(b)

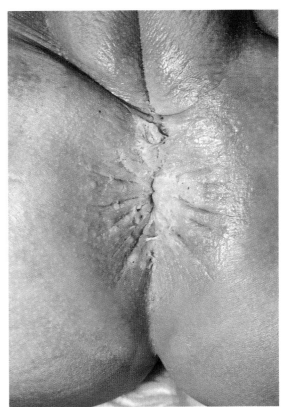

(c)

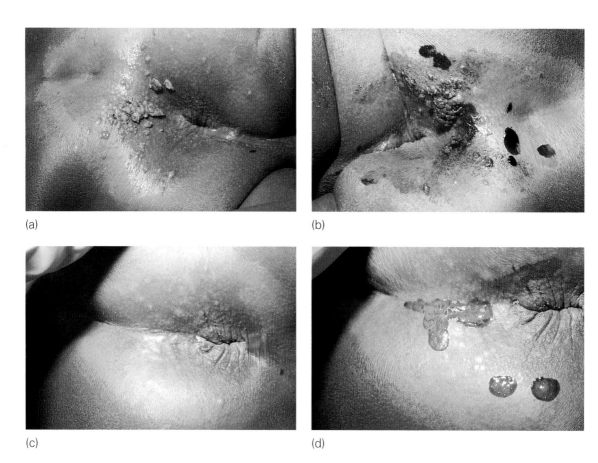

(a)

(b)

(c)

(d)

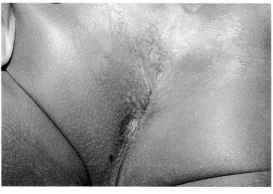

(e)

Figure 7.3

(a) Several solitary and clustered warts of diameter 1–4 mm present in the perianal skin. (b) The appearance of the warts after 25% podophyllin was applied. After drying, a gauze was placed between the buttock cheeks to keep the podophyllin from irritating the apposing skin. (c) One week after initial application of podophyllin, warts are 75% flatter, but some plaque-like lesions remain. (d) Podophyllin is applied for a second treatment in the same manner as the first. (e) One week after the second application, the warts are flatter still. A third applicaton of podophyllin was applied and 1 week later no visible wart remained. The patient remained clear when seen 4 weeks later.

REFERENCES

1. Beutner KR, Ferenczy A. Therapeutic approaches to genital warts. *Am J Med* 1997; **102**: 28–37.
2. Kaplan IW. Condylomata acuminate. *New Orleans Med Surg J* 1942; **94**: 388–90.
3. Romanelli F. Podophyllin. *Clin Toxicol Rev* 1996; **18**. www.maripoisoncenter.com
4. Crowhurst A. *The Weed Cookbook*. New York: Lancer Books, Inc., 1972: 190.
5. Hartwell J. Plants used against cancer. A survey. *Lloydia* 1967; **30**: 379–436.
6. Millspaugh C. *American Medicinal Plants*. New York: Dover Publications, Inc., 1974: 61–4.
7. *Physician's Desk Reference*, 56th edn. Montvale: Medical Economics Company, 2002: 2436–8.
8. von Krogh G. Topical treatment of penile condylomata acuminate with podophyllin, podophyllotoxin and colchicines. *Acta Derm Venereol (Stockh)* 1978; **58**: 163–8.
9. von Krogh G. Penile condylomata acuminate: an experimental model for evaluation of topical self-treatment with 0.5%–1.0% ethanolic preparations of podophyllotoxin for three days. *Sex Transm Dis* 1981; **8**: 179–86.
10. von Krogh G. Topical self-treatment of penile warts with 0.5% podophyllotoxin in ethanol for four or five days. *Sex Transm Dis* 1987; **14**: 135–40.
11. Beutner KR, Conant MA, Friedman-Kien AE et al. Patient-applied podofilox for treatment of genital warts. *Lancet* 1989; **i**: 831–4.
12. Miller RA. Podophyllin. *Int J Dermatol* 1985; 61(5): 338–42.
13. Sullivan M, Friedman M, Hearin JT. *South Med J* 1948; **41**: 336–7.
14. Ferguson LR, Pearson A. Chromosomal changes in Chinese hamster AA8 cells caused by podophyllin, a common treatment for genital warts. *Mut Res* 1992; **266**: 231–9.
15. *Physician's Desk Reference*, 55th edn. Montvale: Medical Economics Company, 2001.
16. Filley CM, Graff-Richard NR, Lacy JR, Heitner MA, Earnest MP. Neurologic manifestations of podophyllin toxicity. *Neurology* 1982; **32**: 308–11.
17. Wade TR, Ackerman AB. The effects of resin of podophyllin on condyloma acuminatum. *Am J Dermatopathol* 1984; **6**: 109–22.
18. Vaughan JT, Montes DF, Bembibre A, Blaquier PC. Condylomata acuminate. *J Cutan Pathol* 1976; **3**: 244–5.
19. Bunney MH, Nolan MW, Williams DA. An assessment of methods of treating viral warts by comparative treatment trials based on a standard design. *Br J Dermatol* 1976; **94**: 667–79.
20. von Krogh G. Topical treatment of penile condylomata acuminate with podophyllin, podophyllotoxin and colchicines. A comparative study. *Acta Derm Venereol (Stockh)* 1978; **58**: 163–8.
21. Simmons PD. Podophyllin 10% and 25% in the treatment of ano-genital warts. A comparative double-blind study. *Br J Vener Dis* 1981; **57**: 208–9.
22. Bashi SA. Cryotherapy versus podophyllin in the treatment of genital warts. *Int J Dermatol* 1985; **24**: 535–6.
23. Jensen SL. Comparison of podophyllin application with simple surgical excision in clearance and recurrence of perianal condylomata acuminata. *Lancet* 1985; **ii**: 1146–8.
24. Lim KB, Lee CT, Koh YL, Yeo WL, Tan T. Self-application of podophyllin resin for penile condylomata acuminate. *Ann Acad Med Singapore* 1987; **16**: 167–9.
25. von Krogh G. Topical self-treatment of penile warts with 0.5% podophyllotoxin in ethanol for four or five days. *Sex Transm Dis* 1987; **14**: 135–40.
26. Lassus A. Comparison of podophyllotoxin and podophyllin in treatment of genital warts. *Lancet* 1987; **ii**: 512–13.
27. Huwyler T, Gutling M, Panizzon R. Experiences with podophyllotoxin in the treatment of condylomata acuminate. *Schweiz Rundsch Med Prax* 1989; **78**: 186–90.

28. Stone KM, Becker TM, Hadgu A, Kraus SJ. Treatment of external genital warts: a randomized clinical trial comparing podophyllin, cryotherapy, and electrodesiccation. *Genitourin Med* 1990; **66**: 16–19.

29. Kirby P, Dunne A, King DH, Corey L. Double-blind randomized clinical trial of self-administered podofilox solution versus vehicle in the treatment of genital warts. *Am J Med* 1990; **88**: 465–9.

30. Baker DA, Douglas JM Jr, Buntin DM, Micha JP, Beutner KR, Patsner B. Topical podofilox for the treatment of condylomata acuminate in women. *Obstet Gynecol* 1990; **76**: 656–9.

31. Greenberg MD, Rutledge LH, Reid R, Berman NR, Precop SL, Elswick RK Jr. A double-blind, randomized trial of 0.5% podofilox and placebo for the treatment of genital warts in women. *Obstet Gynecol* 1991; **77**: 735–9.

32. von Krogh G, Hellberg D. Self-treatment using a 0.5% podophyllotoxin cream of external genital condylomata acuminate in women. A placebo-controlled, double-blind study. *Sex Transm Dis* 1992; **19**: 170–4.

33. Syed TA, Lundin S. Topical treatment of penile condylomata acuminate with podophyllotoxin 0.3% solution, 0.3% cream and 0.15% cream. A comparative open study. *Dermatology* 1993; **187**: 30–3.

34. Syed TA, Lundin S, Ahmad SA. Topical 0.3% and 0.5% podophyllotoxin cream for self-treatment of condylomata acuminate in women. A placebo-controlled, double-blind study. *Dermatology* 1994; **189**: 142–5.

35. von Krogh G, Szpak E, Andersson M, Bergelin I. Self-treatment using 0.25%–0.50% podophyllotoxin-ethanol solutions against penile condylomata acuminate: a placebo-controlled comparative study. *Genitourin Med* 1994; **70**: 105–9.

36. Bonnez W, Elswick RK Jr, Bailey-Farchione A et al. Efficacy and safety of 0.5% podofilox solution in the treatment and suppression of anogenital warts. *Am J Med* 1994; **96**: 420–5.

37. Aynaud O, Tranbaloc P. Treatment of external ano-genital condylomata with 0.5% podophyllotoxin. *Contracept Fertil Sex* 1995; **23**: 127–30.

38. Hellberg D, Svarrer T, Nilsson S, Valentin J. Self-treatment of female external genital warts with 0.5% podophyllotoxin cream (Condyline) vs weekly applications of 20% podophyllin solution. *Int J STD AIDS* 1995; **6**: 257–61.

39. Strand A, Brinkeborn RM, Siboulet A. Topical treatment of genital warts in men, an open study of podophyllotoxin cream compared with solution. *Genitourin Med* 1995; **71**: 387–90.

40. Petersen CS, Agner t, Ottevanger V, Larsen J, Ravnborg L. A single-blind study of podophyllotoxin cream 0.5% and podophyllotoxin solution 0.5% in male patients with genital warts. *Genitourin Med* 1995; **71**: 391–2.

41. Claesson U, Lassus A, Happonen H, Hogstrom L, Siboulet A. Topical treatment of venereal warts: a comparative open study of podophyllotoxin cream versus solution. *Int J STD AIDS* 1996; **7**: 429–34.

42. Tyring S, Edwards L, Cherry LK et al. Safety and efficacy of 0.5% podofilox gel in the treatment of anogenital warts. *Arch Dermatol* 1998; **134**: 33–8.

43. Longstaff E, von Krogh G. Condyloma eradication: self-therapy with 0.15–0.5% podophyllotoxin versus 20–25% podophyllin preparations – an integrated safety assessment. *Regul Toxicol Pharmacol* 2001; **33**: 117–37.

44. von Krogh G, Longstaff E. Podophyllin office therapy against condyloma should be abandoned. *Sex Transm Infect* 2001; **77**: 409–12.

45. Mohanty KC. The cost effectiveness of treatment of genital warts with podophyllotoxin. *Int J STD AIDS* 1994; **5**: 253–6.

46. Langley PC, Tyring SK, Smith MH. The cost effectiveness of patient-applied versus provider-administered intervention strategies for the treatment of external genital warts. *Am J Manag Care* 1999; **5**: 69–77.

8 Other home therapies

Fareedah Goodwin and Robert T Brodell

Cimetidine • Retinoid therapy • Heat therapy • Homeopathy • References

For centuries patients have utilized a variety of home remedies to treat warts. Some of the superstitious 'curing' therapies include rubbing a dusty toad on the wart, rubbing a used washcloth over the wart then burying it in the hope that the wart will disappear as the cloth rots, and rubbing a cut potato on the wart and then throwing the potato over a fence.[1] Although scientifically these remedies seem quite foolish, the public often sees them as inexpensive options with minimal side effects that allow them to avoid expensive physicians or offer hope when allopathic medicine fails.

Therapies that will be discussed in this chapter include cimetidine, retinoids, homeopathy, and heat therapy. Some of these agents have been tested for their effectiveness in treating warts, whereas others are supported by very little scientific evidence. With further study, these agents may prove to be useful alternative or adjunctive modes of therapy for warts.

simplex, and Epstein–Barr virus infections. In addition it has immunomodulatory effects, demonstrated in the treatment of mucocutaneous candidiasis and common variable immunodeficiency. More recently, it has been evaluated for the treatment of multiple recalcitrant viral warts.[2]

Basic science

Cimetidine has immunomodulatory effects that are not completely understood. At high doses (30–40 mg/kg per day), cimetidine inhibits the stimulatory effects of histamine on suppressor T lymphocytes. This inhibition of suppressor T cells occurs at the same time that cimetidine increases lymphocytic proliferation. Thus, cell-mediated immunity of the host is augmented in a non-specific manner to enhance defenses against papillomavirus infections.[3]

CIMETIDINE

Historical aspects

Cimetidine has been used as alternative therapy for a variety of infectious skin diseases, including herpes zoster, herpes

Clinical evidence

Both open-label and placebo-controlled studies have been carried out to determine the efficacy of cimetidine for the treatment of warts. An open-label study by Glass and Solomon[4] enrolled 20 adult patients who had recalcitrant warts (warts present for 2 or more years despite treatment with at least two prior treatment regimens). Each participant in the study was treated with cimetidine 30–40 mg/kg per day for 3 months. Of the 18 patients who completed the study, 16 (84%) reported either complete resolution of their warts or dramatic improvement of their lesions. The patients who did not report improvement had been given the lower dosage of 30 mg/kg per day. Therefore, this study concluded that cimetidine was a safe and beneficial therapy for difficult warts if given at higher doses. Another open-label study done by Orlow et al[2] had similar results.

A double-masked, placebo-controlled study by Karabulut et al[5] had quite different results. In their study, 54 patients with recalcitrant warts (a wart for at least 6 months and refractory to other therapies) were selected. Patients were randomly assigned to either the cimetidine or the placebo group. The patients were not permitted to use any other systemic or topical medication during, and for at least 4 weeks before starting, the study. As long as no new lesions appeared, the patients were continued on their therapy for a total of 12 weeks. A total of 43 patients completed the study: 27 in the cimetidine group and 16 in the placebo group. Of the patients receiving the cimetidine 37% reported complete resolution of their warts, whereas 25% of the patients receiving the placebo reported such results. As the sample was so small, there was no significant difference in response to therapy between the cimetidine and placebo groups ($P > 0.05$). Therefore, they concluded that cimetidine was no better than placebo in treating warts. However, in this study all the patients with flat warts were found to have complete resolution of their lesions. This suggests that cimetidine may have a selective beneficial effect on flat warts. Of course, further research is needed to substantiate these benefits. A placebo-controlled study by Yilmaz et al[6] had similar negative results.

In summary, the literature is not conclusive about the efficacy of cimetidine in treating warts. The improvement noted in several open-label studies may represent a placebo effect. As the evidence supporting the use of cimetidine is based on small open-label studies, and its utility is refuted by small randomized, placebo-controlled studies, any recommendation for its use must rest on the opinions of experts in the field, who are themselves divided. It is judged to be level V according to our Modified Evidence-based Medicine System (see Chapter 19).

Adverse effects

Adverse effects reported by patients in the cimetidine studies were unusual, the most common complaints being gastrointestinal symptoms. Patients should not take phenytoin or theophylline while using cimetidine because of adverse drug–drug interactions secondary to cimetidine's action on cytochrome P450 enzymes.

Cost–benefit considerations

Cimetidine is a relatively inexpensive alternative treatment for warts. For a 60-kg person, a full 3-month course of 'high-dose' cimetidine 40 mg/kg would cost $US153. This is a rather inexpensive form of therapy requiring few visits to the doctor's surgery. However, in the absence of clear-cut benefits, this low cost does not offer real value.

RETINOID THERAPY
Historical aspects

Retinoids have been used in dermatology since the early part of the twentieth century.

The anti-keratotic properties of vitamin A have been known since 1932. In 1949, Studer and Frey demonstrated that large oral doses of a certain vitamin A derivative could decrease the rate of epidermal proliferation.[7] The use of retinoids in the treatment of warts was first reported in the early 1970s.[8]

Basic science

Retinoids have been utilized for the treatment of warts because they alter keratinization and change the microenvironment of differentiated keratinocytes. As the papillomavirus replicates in these differentiated cells, a change in their environment could, in theory, make successful replication less likely. In addition, moderate doses of isotretinoin and etretinate have been shown to cause a transient increase in natural killer cell activity, which suggests that retinoids have immunomodulatory effects.[9] Retinoids also induce an irritant dermatitis that may accelerate the clearing of warts through non-specific inflammatory effects.[10]

Clinical evidence

An open-label trial done by Naik et al[11] studied intralesional injection of vitamin A combined with suggestive psychotherapy; 53 patients completed the study. The average number of injections for each wart was five, and the average time to clearing was 7 weeks. At the end of the study, 43 patients had complete clearing of their warts, which was a cure rate of 81.2%. One especially interesting finding was noted – warts that developed more severe degrees of inflammation around the vitamin A injection sites were associated with better response and shorter duration of therapy. There may be a relationship between the vitamin A-induced inflammation and wart clearance.

In an open-label study by de Bersaques, the results were not favorable[12]; 50 patients were recruited for the study, and all their plantar warts were treated with a 2% vitamin A acid ointment under occlusion. At the end of the trial, only 17 of the 50 patients were reported to be wart free.

In a case study by Boyle et al[13] oral etretinate was utilized for the treatment of warts in a 22-year-old man with sarcoidosis. The patient had rapidly developing warts on his face, neck, and palms after prednisolone was used to treat his sarcoidosis. One month after beginning oral etretinate, the hyperkeratosis of his hands was reduced and the warts on his face had disappeared. Unfortunately, the warts recurred after stopping the etretinate therapy.

In a case study by Goihman-Yahr,[10] an 8-year-old girl who had multiple plane warts of 2 months' duration over her cheeks was treated with tretinoin cream on one cheek and 3% salicylic acid preparation on the other. Two weeks after treatment, the cheek that had been treated with tretinoin had developed an irritant reaction, whereas the other cheek had no reaction. A week after the inflammation subsided on the tretinoin-treated cheek, no plane warts remained.

Based on this evidence, retinoids may well have some limited value in the treatment of warts and, therefore, would be classified as a level V according to our Modified Evidence-based Medicine System (Chapter 19).

Adverse effects

Topical retinoids and intralesional retinoids can cause local irritation. Systemic retinoids cause dryness and flaking; they must be avoided in pregnant women and carefully used in women of childbearing potential. In the case of 13-*cis*-retinoic acid, pregnancy must be prevented while the patient is on the medication systemically and for 1 month thereafter. In the case of acetretin, patients taking this medicine should probably never get pregnant because there is a long-term risk of birth defects even after women have stopped the medication. Liver inflammation, increased triglycerides, pseudotumor cerebri, and hyperostoses may also occur.

Cost–benefit considerations

The price of topical tretinoin ranges from $US48 to $US54 for 45-gram tubes. In the absence of proven efficacy, these costs have little significance. The cost of a single 25 mg tablet of Acetretin is $14.53. A 30 day supply (one daily) would cost $435.90.

HEAT THERAPY

Historical aspects

Heat therapy had its beginnings in veterinary medicine for the treatment of various benign and malignant conditions, e.g. it was studied in mouse melanoma. The ability to use localized heat to control superficial tissue destruction has made this mode of therapy an interesting alternative to traditional wart treatment.

Basic science

Heat therapy acts by injuring the tissue occupied by the wart. As it is thought that the diseased tissue will be more sensitive to the effects of elevated temperature, it may also heal more slowly after thermal injury. Furthermore, inflammation induced in tissue may be important.

Clinical evidence

Stern and Levine[14] performed a placebo-controlled study, using heat therapy, in the treatment of warts; 13 patients were enrolled with a total of 46 warts. The warts were anesthetized with 1% lidocaine, and then were treated with either localized heat produced by a radiofrequency current or by a placebo device that was identical in appearance to the heating device. Each heat-treated wart received one to four 30- to 60-second treatments at 50°C. Of the 29 treated warts, 25 (86%) regressed completely; of the 17 control warts, 7 (41%) resolved during the study. It was concluded that localized heat therapy could induce regression of hand warts. We classify heat therapy as level V according to our Modified Evidence-based Medicine System (Chapter 19) based on a single small open-label study and anecdotes. This is insufficient evidence to recommend this modality in clinical practice.

Adverse effects

Heat therapy has inherent risks. Application of localized heat to the tissue around the wart can cause erythema, edema, crusting, and scarring. However, in the study reviewed above, most patients complained of only mild discomfort during treatment.

Cost–benefit considerations

The heat therapy device studied requires visits to the doctor's surgery and is performed by a physician, making it moderately expensive. Heat therapy can be used very inexpensively if one substitutes the radiofrequency heating device used in the aforementioned study for a heating apparatus that can be used at home, such as a hot-water bottle. It is doubtful, however, that home therapy with low-technology devices could induce sustained temperatures of 50°C for 30–60 min. In the absence of proven benefit, cost–benefit analysis is difficult.

HOMEOPATHY

Historical aspects

Homeopathy, which means to 'treat like with like', has become more and more popular as people are inclined to seek 'natural' and alternative remedies for various ailments. Homeopathy was first popularized in the medical profession in the sixteenth and seventeenth centuries and was called the 'Doctrine of Signatures'. This name alluded to the belief that God had imprinted certain curative 'signs' in various plants. Plant extracts are diluted thousands of times so that the original molecules of the substance are not present, but the memory of the substance is somehow imprinted in the water solvent. However, after the onset of the 'Scientific Revolution', homeopathy was largely relegated to folk practice. Now it seems to be reappearing in the medical community.[15]

Basic science

Although homeopathy is based on the idea that 'like cures like', there has been no scientific validation of this concept or any pathophysiologic basis for effectiveness beyond the placebo effect.

Clinical evidence

A randomized, double-blind trial of homeopathic versus placebo therapy in the treatment of warts was performed by Kainz et al[16]. In this study 60 children were enrolled, all of whom had common warts on the hands. Half were randomly selected to receive one of 10 homeopathic preparations, whereas the other half received a placebo. Some of the substances used in the preparations included Calcium carbonicum and Sulfur. Reduction of the wart by at least 50% was considered a positive response to therapy. At the end of the study, nine of the 30 patients receiving the homeopathic preparation had responded, whereas seven of the 30 patients receiving the placebo had reduction in wart size. Five patients in the homeopathy group had complete cure of warts, and one in the placebo group had complete resolution. It was concluded that the homeopathic preparation was not superior to placebo. Supportive homeopathy in the treatment of warts is rated level V according to our Modified Evidence-based Medicine System (Chapter 19).

Adverse effects

As far as homeopathy is concerned, it is difficult to determine the potential for adverse reactions as there is no Food and Drug Administration regulation of these remedies in the USA, although we would guess that side effects are probably rare using agents 'diluted' homeopathically till the original active molecules are not present.

Cost–benefit considerations

Homeopathic remedies are generally used at home and can be inexpensive or expensive to purchase. Unless a benefit can be shown using homeopathic approaches, cost–benefit comparison with effective therapies is not possible.

Summary of these 'alternative' modalities

Of the above alternative therapies for wart treatment, there is a modicum of evidence to support the use of retinoids, heat therapy, and cimetidine. In the absence of standardized protocols with proven effectiveness, none of these is recommended for routine use, although they may be helpful in individual patients.

REFERENCES

1. Bolton, Ruth. Nongenital warts: classification and treatment options. *Am Fam Physician* 1991; **6**: 2055.
2. Orlow SJ, Paller A. Cimetidine therapy for multiple viral warts in children. *J Am Acad Dermatol* 1993; **28**: 794–6.
3. Rogers CJ, Gibney MD, Siegfried EC, Harrison BR, Glaser DA. Cimetidine therapy for recalcitrant warts in adults: is it any better than placebo? *J Am Acad Dermatol* 1999; **41**: 123–6.
4. Glass AT, Solomon BA. Cimetidine therapy for recalcitrant warts in adults. *Arch Dermatol* 1996; **132**: 680–2.
5. Karabulut AA, Sahin S, Eksioglu M. Is cimetidine effective for nongenital warts: a double-blind, placebo-controlled study. *Arch Dermatol* 1997; **133**: 533–4.
6. Yilmaz E, Alpsoy E, Basran E. Cimetidine therapy for warts: A placebo-controlled, double-blind study. *J Am Acad Dermatol* 1996; **34**: 1005–7.
7. Stuttgen, G. Historical perspectives of tretinoin. *J Am Acad Dermatol* 1986; **15**: 735–9.
8. Goldfarb MT, Gupta AK, Gupta MA, Sawchuk WS. Office therapy for human papillomavirus infection in nongenital sites. *Dermatol Clin* 1991; **9**: 287–95.
9. Griffiths WAD. Retinoids in the treatment of warts. *Retinoids Today and Tomorrow?* 22–4.
10. Goihman-Yahr, M. Treatment of plane warts by tretinoin-induced irritant reaction (correspondence). *Int J Dermatol* 1994; **33**: 826–7.
11. Naik PVS, Pillai KG, Paily PP. Injection of vitamin-A in the treatment of warts (a clinical trial). *Ind J Dermatol* 1974; **19**: 87–9.
12. De Bersaques J. Vitamin A acid in the topic treatment of plantar warts. *Dermatologica* 1975; **150**: 369–71.
13. Boyle J, Dick DC, Mackie RM. Treatment of extensive virus warts with etretinate (Tigason) in a patient with sarcoidosis. *Clin Exp Dermatol* 1983; **8**: 33–6.
14. Stern P, Levine N. Controlled localized heat therapy in cutaneous warts. *Arch Dermatol* 1992; **128**: 945–7.
15. Whorton JC. Traditions of folk medicine in America. *JAMA* 1987; **257**: 1632–5.
16. Kainz JT, Kozel G, Haidvogl M, Smolle J. Homeopathic versus placebo therapy of children with warts on the hands: a randomized, double-blind clinical trial. *Dermatology* 1997; **193**: 318–20.

Part III
Office-based therapies

9 Liquid nitrogen in the treatment of viral warts

Sandra Marchese Johnson and Jessica Causbie Pillow

Historical aspects • Basic science • Clinical studies • Favored treatment methodology • Course and prognosis • Contraindications to treatment • Case scenarios • References

Cryotherapy (cryosurgery) is the standard therapy for viral warts that are resistant to over-the-counter topical agents, or for large warts where it is anticipated that home therapy will be ineffective. Liquid nitrogen is the substance most frequently employed for cryotherapy of the skin. We limit out discussion of cryotherapy to liquid nitrogen, which is a safe, simple and inexpensive method of wart treatment. Cryotherapy produces minimal scarring and can be performed in both the hospital and the surgery setting. In this chapter, the use of liquid nitrogen cryotherapy for treatment of warts is reviewed.

The development of cryogenic equipment was advanced with the 'complete cryogenic surgical system' designed by Cooper.[3] The system included a cooling cannula, which was vacuum insulated, except at the tip, to allow temperatures as low as −190°C. It also contained a thermocouple located within the cooling tip. Further advances included development of the first hand-held liquid nitrogen device, the Kryospray.[4] Today, cryotherapy of warts is accomplished with a variety of techniques using applicators, probes and sprays.

HISTORICAL ASPECTS

Before liquid nitrogen was readily available, liquid air and liquid oxygen were used as wart-removal refrigerants.[1] The use of liquid nitrogen to treat warts was first documented by Allington in 1950,[2] who used a cotton-tipped applicator dipped in liquid nitrogen. He described the speed and ease of application as well as the minimal pain incurred as a result of treatment. Furthermore, little postoperative care was required, infection was rare and scarring was minimal.

BASIC SCIENCE

Liquid nitrogen has a boiling point of −195.6°C. When applied, liquid nitrogen cools the skin as it evaporates and acts as a heat sink. The treated skin is frozen immediately and the freeze spreads equally in all directions. However, the temperature of the skin is inconsistent within the area treated, with the coldest area being closest to the point of application. The length of freeze also affects the temperature gradient: the slower the freeze, the larger the temperature gradient between treated and untreated skin, i.e. the temperature difference is inversely proportional to the rate of the freeze. Tissue death occurs to benign tissue that is frozen below –20°C. Some providers use a thermocouple to measure the temperature of the treated skin, which leads to increased precision and accuracy. Tissue destruction occurs in two phases, with the first phase comprising intra- and extracellular ice formation. When skin is treated with a fast freeze and a slow thaw, the tissue destruction occurs primarily as a result of intracellular ice formation. Ischemic necrosis, the second phase, occurs because the skin microvasculature is very cryosensitive.[5] Multiple freeze-thaw cycles are more destructive than one cycle, especially for plantar warts.[5,6]

Liquid nitrogen does not kill human papillomavirus.[7] Cryotherapy is therefore considered a destructive modality, and every wart on a patient should be treated when using cryotherapy.

The skin cell that is the most sensitive to cryoinjury is the melanocyte. Hypo- and hyperpigmentation changes are very common after liquid nitrogen therapy, and hair follicles and peripheral nerves are also sensitive to cryoinjury.[5]

As the nerves are cryosensitive, liquid nitrogen therapy can be painful. The pain often limits the treatment in areas with an increased nerve supply such as the digits and the genitals. There have been many attempts to diminish the pain associated with cryotherapy, and some success has been shown with topical and intralesional anesthesia.[8]

CLINICAL STUDIES

Although there are few supporting data, home use of salicylic acid wart paint is often used as an adjunct to cryotherapy. In one trial, combined use of salicylic acid paint and liquid nitrogen produced a cure rate of 78% versus 69% for patients treated with liquid nitrogen

alone and 67% for patients treated with salicylic acid paint alone.[9]

In general, warts do not require preparation before cryotherapy, although plantar warts tend to be more calloused than warts in other locations, and paring before cryotherapy often enhances their clearance. It was noted in the 1960s that the excess keratin overlying plantar warts acts as an insulator to the freezing temperatures encountered during cryotherapy. Liquid nitrogen is more effective for plantar warts when combined with aggressive paring of the excess keratin before treatment,[10] and complete cure rates of 75–93% can be expected.[11–13]

Cryotherapy is also a practical and effective option in the treatment of genital warts. A controlled study of 64 patients receiving weekly fine-needle cryotherapy reported cure rates of 83% within 4 weeks and 96% after 6 weeks. These results were similar to other methods of treatment. The mean number of treatments to cure was 1.37–4.3, depending on the number of warts present. Generally, larger numbers of warts correlate with increased numbers of treatments. The advantages are that duration of treatment is short and no general anesthesia is necessary. In this study, recurrence rates were not studied.[14]

Traditionally, the interval between treatments of common warts with cryotherapy is 3 weeks. An early study demonstrated that intervals longer than 3 weeks are much less efficacious when cure is measured at 12 weeks.[9] Another study compared 1-, 2- and 3-week intervals and found that the cure rates after 12 treatments were similar in all groups. In this study, the 2-week interval produced cure after almost the same number of treatments as the 3-week interval without increasing departmental workload. This was not true for the weekly treated group, which returned for more follow-up visits than the other groups. The researchers concluded that a more rapid cure might be obtained by treating more frequently than 3 weeks. However, more frequent treat-

Table 9.1 Comparison of clinical trials using liquid nitrogen versus other treatment methods in the eradication of common warts

Treatment method	Type of trial	Number of patients	Percentage cure rates	Reference
LN2 vs salicylic acid and lactic acid (SAL) vs both LN2 and SAL	RCT	294	Percentage cure rates 69 vs 67 vs 78	9
LN2 and SAL with paring vs without paring	RCT	400	46 vs 50 all warts; 75 vs 39 plantar warts; no benefit to continue LN2 after 3 months	11
Liquid nitrogen spray vs cotton-wool bud	CCT	363	44 vs 47 cure at 3 months	16
LN2 at 1-, 2- and 3-week intervals	RCT	225	After 3 months: 43 vs 37 vs 26 cure. After 12 treatments: 43 vs 48 vs 44 cure	15
LN2 at 3- vs 4-week intervals	RCT	72	75 vs 40	9
LN2: 1 freeze vs 2 freezes	RCT	207	57 vs 62 cure of all people who completed protocol, 41 vs 65 of plantar warts	6
LN2 vs control	CCT	64	96 vs 45	14
LN2 vs acyclovir vs placebo	CCT	47	9 vs 39 vs 28	17
LN2 vs TCA	RCT	130 men	88 vs 81	18
LN2 vs TCA	RCT	86	86 vs 70	19
LN2 vs electrosurgery	RCT	42	No difference	20
LN2 with IFNα_{2a} vs LN2 with placebo	RCT	60	61 vs 68	21
LN2 vs podophyllin vs electrodessication	RCT	450	79 vs 41 vs 94	22
LN2 vs mumps skin test antigen vs candida skin test antigen	RCT	115	57 vs 71 vs 88	23
LN2 vs pulsed dye laser vs cantharidin	RCT	194 warts	No difference	24

LN2, liquid nitrogen cryotherapy; SAL, salicylic acid; RCT, randomized clinical trial; CCT, controlled clinical trial; TCA, trichloroacetic acid.

ments limit the time for healing between applications, and therefore adverse events such as blistering and pain are more common. The report did not mention whether or not scarring or pigment changes were more common in the weekly treated group.[15] Regardless of

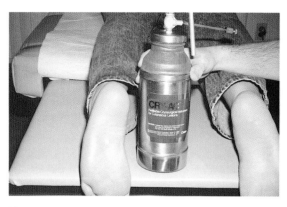

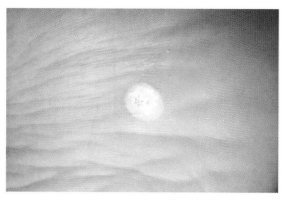

Figure 9.1
A cryogen spray canister commonly used to apply liquid nitrogen to warts.

Figure 9.2
The appearance of a plantar wart immediately after liquid nitrogen was applied for 25 seconds. The white frozen skin highlights thrombosed capillaries within the wart.

interval, cure is unlikely with fewer than three treatments.[9]

If continued for more than 3 months, cryotherapy becomes less effective, and it is recommended to change therapies if there is limited improvement after 3 months of treatments.[11] For further comparison of liquid nitrogen versus other treatment methods in the eradication of common warts, see Table 9.1.

The strength of the recommendations supporting the use of liquid nitrogen cryotherapy in the treatment of warts can be estimated using evidence-based medicine techniques. As various papers were reviewed, many of which were well-designed, randomized controlled studies, the recommendations included in this chapter for the treatment of common and genital warts with liquid nitrogen cryotherapy are based on level 1 evidence (see Chapter 19).

FAVOURED TREATMENT METHODOLOGY

Liquid nitrogen is commonly applied with an applicator or a spray. An applicator is prepared by unwrapping a cotton ball and then wrapping this cotton around the cotton end of a Q-tip, forming a pear-shaped applicator, which serves as a reservoir for liquid nitrogen. The cotton tip is dipped into a container of liquid nitrogen and applied directly to the wart. A separate applicator should be used for each patient. As the applicator is tipped upward, more liquid nitrogen is delivered to the site and a broader area is frozen. When treating with a canister to produce a spray (Figure 9.1), the device is held at a 90° angle just above the wart.[26] With either method, a typical procedure entails freezing a wart for 10–30 seconds with a 1- to 2-mm rim of white frozen tissue surrounding the wart (Figure 9.2). This is followed by a thaw time of 20–30 seconds. Sometimes, two cycles of freezing and thawing are performed to achieve maximum tissue destruction, although for common warts away from the palms or soles and for genital warts, we generally use a single freeze. Repeat treatments are given every 2–4 weeks until resolution or 3 months of therapy.[9,11,15,27]

Paring of excess hyperkeratosis is recommended before initial cryotherapy for the plantar aspect of the foot and just prior to

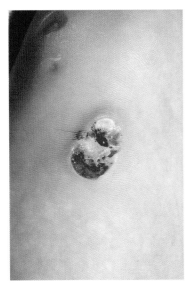

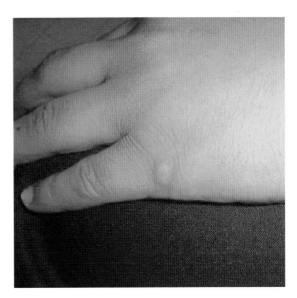

Figure 9.3
The base of an unroofed blister 1 week after liquid nitrogen cryotherapy, with two areas of persistent wart showing scalloped edges. Additional treatment is required.

Figure 9.4
This 5 × 6 mm area of hypopigmentation was present 1 month after a wart was treated with liquid nitrogen. No evidence of wart remains.

subsequent treatments (Figure 9.3). The authors also use two freeze-thaw cycles when treating areas with excess hyperkeratosis.

COURSE AND PROGNOSIS

To avoid high levels of frustration, the patient should be instructed about the immediate post-treatment course and long-term outcomes after cryotherapy (Table 9.2). The patient will feel a burning sensation on application of liquid nitrogen, which intensifies as the lesion thaws. The pain will lessen over 2–3 hours and then disappear.[1] Local erythema and edema develop immediately after treatment. After several hours, a blister may develop. After about 3 days, ischaemic necrosis begins and a crust or scab forms. Re-epithelialization occurs with little or no resultant scar formation (Figure 9.4).[29]

An average of 3.1–5.5 treatments are needed to cure warts. Percentage cure varies widely among studies, and recurrence rates have been speculated to be caused primarily by incomplete treatment.[9,15] It has been reported that sex, age, prior treatment and number of warts per individual do not negatively affect the cure rate with cryotherapy. However, the larger the diameter of the wart or the longer the duration of the wart, the less likely the chance for cure. Plane warts are also more resistant to cryotherapy than other wart types; whether this is the result of the viral type or the location is not clear.[11]

CONTRAINDICATIONS TO TREATMENT

Patients who should avoid cryosurgery include those with areas of poor circulation

Table 9.2 Patient education sheet

What is cryosurgery?

Cryosurgery is a procedure in which abnormal body tissues are destroyed by exposure to extremely cold temperatures.

How do I prepare for cryosurgery?

There is no special preparation for cryosurgery. It is a simple procedure that is done in a short time in your healthcare provider's surgery.

What happens during the procedure?

Your healthcare provider will use a probe, spray tool or cotton-tipped applicator dipped in liquid nitrogen to treat the affected areas. A very cold gas, usually liquid nitrogen, is applied to freeze the wart. You will feel a burning and stinging sensation while the area freezes and then thaws. Although the procedure may cause some discomfort, an anesthetic is rarely needed. The length of time the wart is frozen depends on the size and type of the lesion. For some lesions, the procedure works best if the tissue is frozen quickly, allowed to thaw and then frozen again.

What happens after the procedure?

A small blister will usually form. The blister will later become a scab or a crust. Healing usually occurs over 7–10 days. Warts often need to be treated more than once. Your healthcare provider will tell you how often you need to be checked for recurrence or re-treatment, even if the warts appear to have cleared. You will need a follow-up visit to check healing and to see if tiny amounts of abnormal tissue remain.

What are the benefits of cryosurgery?

Cryosurgery is very effective and is less expensive than other treatments. It can be done in your healthcare provider's surgery and anesthesia is usually not necessary.

What are the risks associated with cryosurgery?

The risks include: discoloration of the treated area, which can be either light or dark; damaged hair and sweat glands in the treated area; minor scarring and recurrence. If warts recur, reschedule an appointment with your healthcare provider for re-treatment.

When should I call the doctor?

Call your doctor's office if:

- The treated area is bleeding or not healing 2–3 weeks after surgery
- The lesions reappear
- The treated area looks infected

Adapted from Clinical Reference Systems.[28]

because these areas may form ulcers and heal slowly following treatment. Patients with the following conditions are inclined to have increased adverse effects after cryotherapy: macroglobulinemia, immuno-proliferative neoplasms, active collagen vascular disease, active ulcerative colitis, high serum cryoglobulin levels, subacute bacterial endocarditis, syphilis, Epstein–Barr virus infection, cytomegalovirus infection or chronic hepatitis B, and patients on high-dose steroid medication. In these patients, pre-testing an area of the skin and shortening the duration of freeze are recommended.[29]

CASE REPORTS

Case 1

A 20-year-old man presented with a 4-month history of a painful plaque on the plantar aspect of his left foot. Over-the-counter wart therapies proved unsuccessful. On physical examination a 9-mm hyperkeratotic plaque with central punctate black pinpoint macules was found in a healthy man. The diagnosis of plantar warts led to a discussion of various treatment options with the patient; he opted for treatment with cryotherapy. The wart was pared with a 15 blade to remove excess hyperkeratosis. Liquid nitrogen was applied to the wart using a cryogen spray canister for 10 seconds. The wart and a 3-mm rim of normal skin were encompassed in the treated area. The tissue thawed and liquid nitrogen was reapplied for 10 more seconds. The time of freeze for each treatment was 10 seconds. Every 3 weeks the patient was re-evaluated and treated as needed. Over-the-counter therapy with daily application of salicylic acid was used at home in between visits to the surgery. The wart resolved after four visits (12 weeks).

Case 2

A 16-year-old girl presents with two 'ugly' growths on her right index finger, which bother the mother and father more than the patient. They have been present for 3 weeks and no treatment has been used. On physical examination, this healthy teenage girl has two 4-mm diameter verrucous papules on her right index finger. The diagnosis of verruca vulgaris (common warts) is made. Treatment options were discussed with the patient and her parents, and treatment with liquid nitrogen cryotherapy was chosen. The risks and benefits were explored and signed informed consent was obtained. Liquid nitrogen was applied to the warts and a 3-mm rim of normal skin for a total freeze time of 10 seconds. The patient returned in 3 weeks for re-evaluation and treatment with resolution without visible scarring was achieved after two treatments.

REFERENCES

1. Cooper SM, Dawber RPR. The history of cryosurgery. *J R Soc Med* 2001; **94**: 196–200.
2. Allington H. Liquid nitrogen in the treatment of skin diseases. *Calif Med* 1950; **72**: 153–5.
3. Cooper IS. Cryogenic surgery: A new method of destruction or extirpation of benign or malignant tissue. *N Engl J Med* 1963; **268**: 743–9.
4. Zacarian S. Cryogenics: The cryolesion and the pathogenesis of cryonecrosis. In: Zacarian SA, ed. *Cryosurgery for Skin Cancer and Cutaneous Disorders*. St Louis: Mosby, 1985: 1–30.
5. Wilkes TDI, Fraunfelder FT. Principles of cryosurgery. *Ophthal Surg* 1979; **8**: 21–9.
6. Berth-Jones J, Bourke J, Eglitis H, et al. Value of a second freeze cycle in cryotherapy of common warts. *Br J Dermatol* 1994; **131**: 883–6.

7. Jones SK, Darville JM. Transmission of virus particles by cryotherapy and multi-use caustic pencils: a problem to dermatologists? *Br J Dermatol* 1989; **121**: 481–6.

8. Menter A, Black-Noller G, Riendeau LA, Monti KL. The use of EMLA cream and 1% lidocaine in men for relief of pain associated with the removal of genital warts by cryotherapy. *J Am Acad Dermatol* 1997; **37**: 96–100.

9. Bunney MH, Nolan MW, Williams DA. An assessment of methods treating viral warts by comparative treatment trials based on a standard design. *Br J Dermatol* 1976; **94**: 667–79.

10. Kee CE. Liquid nitrogen cryotherapy. *Arch Dermatol* 1967; **96**: 198–203.

11. Berth-Jones J, Hutchinson PE. Modern treatment of warts: cure rates at 3 and 6 months. *Br J Dermatol* 1992; **127**: 262–5.

12. Buckley D. Cryosurgery treatment of plantar warts. *Irish Med J* 2000; **93**: 140–3.

13. Hewitt WR Jr. Liquid nitrogen treatment of hand and plantar warts. *J Am Coll Health* 1992; **40**: 288–9.

14. Damstra RJ, van Vloten WA. Cryotherapy in the treatment of condyloma acuminata: a controlled study of 64 patients. *J Dermatol Surg Oncol* 1991; **17**: 273–6.

15. Bourke JF, Berth-Jones J, Hutchinson PE. Cryotherapy of common viral warts at intervals of 1, 2, and 3 weeks. *Br J Dermatol* 1995; **132**: 433–6.

16. Ahemed J, Agarwal S, Ilchyshen A et al. Liquid nitrogen cryotherapy of common warts: cryo-spray vs. cotton wool bud. *Br J Dermatol* 2001; **144**: 1006–9.

17. Gibson JR, Harvery SG, Barth J et al. A comparison of acyclovir cream versus Placebo cream versus liquid nitrogen in the treatment of viral plantar warts. *Dermatologica* 1984; **168**: 178–81.

18. Godley MJ, Bradbeer CS, Gellan M et al. Cryotherapy compared with trichloroacetic acid in treating genital warts. *Genitourin Med* 1987; **63**: 390–2.

19. Abdullah AN, Walzman M, Wade A. Treatment of external genital warts comparing cryotherapy (liquid nitrogen) and trichloroacetic acid. *Sex Transm Dis* 1993; **20**: 344–5.

20. Simmons PD, Langlet F, Tin RN. Cryotherapy versus electrosurgery in the treatment of genital warts. *Br J Vener Dis* 1981; **57**: 273–4.

21. Handley JM, Horner T, Maw RD et al. Subcutaneous interferon alpha 2a combined with cryotherapy vs cryotherapy alone in the treatment of primary anogenital warts: a randomised observer blind placebo controlled study. *Genitourin Med* 1991; **67**: 297–302.

22. Stone KM, Becker TM, Hadgu A et al. Treatment of external genital warts: a randomised clinical trial comparing podophyllin, cryotherapy, and electrodessication. *Genitourin Med* 1990; **66**: 16–19.

23. Johnson SM, Roberson PK, Horn TD. Intralesional injection of mumps or candida antigens: a novel immunotherapy for warts. *Arch Dermatol* 2001; **137**: 451–5.

24. Robson KJ, Cunningham NM, Kruzan KL et al. Pulsed-dye laser versus conventional therapy in the treatment of warts: a prospective randomized trial. *J Am Acad Dermatol* 2000; **43**: 275–80.

25. Jester DM. Cryotherapy of dermal abnormalities. *Prim Care* 1997; **24**: 269–80.

26. Johnson SM, Brodell RT. Warts: A guide to their removal. *Consultant* 1999; **39**: 253–66.

27. Women's Health Advisor. Patient education handout: outpatient cryosurgery. Clinical Reference Systems 2001; www.mdconsult.com.

28. Hocutt JE. Skin cryosurgery for the family physician. *Am Fam Physician* 1993; **48**: 445–52.

10 Bleomycin

*Marla Lindsey Wirges, Charles M Davis and
Sandra Marchese Johnson*

**Historical aspects • Basic science • Clinical evidence • Case report •
Favored treatment methodology • Adverse effects • Course and
prognosis • Evidence-based medicine • References**

Bleomycin has been used in the treatment of warts since the early 1970s. The exact mechanism by which bleomycin leads to resolution of warts is not understood, although damage to viral DNA and antiviral effects are thought to play a primary role. Most clinical trials demonstrated significant benefit from intralesional bleomycin injections, but others did not and this led to controversy about its true effectiveness.[1,2] Treatment is generally well tolerated by patients.

HISTORICAL ASPECTS

Bleomycin was discovered as an anti-tumor antimicrobial in 1965 by Umezawa and colleagues.[3] It was isolated as a fermentation product from the soil fungus *Streptomyces verticellus*. One of the earliest clinical uses of bleomycin was to treat squamous cell carcinomas of the head and neck.[4] Today, bleomycin is commonly used intralesionally to treat warts and systemically to treat lymphomas, testicular tumors, and squamous cell carcinomas of the cervix, head and neck, and lungs.

BASIC SCIENCE

Bleomycin is a water-soluble polypeptide mixture with antineoplastic, antibiotic and antiviral properties. The core of the bleomycin molecule is a complex metal-binding structure. Attached to the core is a tripeptide chain and a terminal dithiazole carboxylic acid that binds to DNA.[5] The commercially available mixture of bleomycin sulfate, or Blenoxane, is composed of 11 different glycopeptides.[6] The majority of these peptides are bleomycin A2 and bleomycin B2, which differ only in their terminal amine.

The antineoplastic effect of bleomycin is related to its ability to bind to DNA and generate free radicals. This causes oxidative damage to nucleotides and leads to single- and double-stranded chromosomal breaks. Bleomycin also inhibits DNA synthesis and causes accumulation of cells in the G2 phase of the cell cycle. To a lesser extent it inhibits RNA and protein synthesis. Similarly, bleomycin is thought to exert antiviral effects by binding to the viral genome and preventing replication.

Although the exact mechanism by which bleomycin leads to resolution of warts is unclear, its damaging effects on DNA and antiviral properties are assumed to have a primary role. Several studies have elucidated specific effects of bleomycin on warts. Templeton et al[7] used light microscopy and immunofluorescence to examine normal skin after injection with bleomycin. They found expression and upregulation of cell adhesion molecules on endothelial cells and activation antigens on keratinocytes. A neutrophilic infiltrate was consistently present. This suggests that cytokine secretion and cellular immune response also have a role to play in wart resolution with bleomycin. This is supported by a study by Sobh et al[8] which showed that immunosuppressed renal transplant recipients had decreased efficacy with bleomycin (36.6%) when compared with non-transplant patients (59%).[8] James et al[9] suggested another theory after finding apoptotic keratinocytes high in the epidermis of warts 48 hours after injection with bleomycin. They concluded that bleomycin must have a direct toxic effect on keratinocytes, leading to biochemical changes and cell death in addition to its effect on DNA.

Bleomycin is degraded by a specific hydrolase found in various tissues, including the liver, spleen and bone marrow red cells.[8] This hydrolase is notably decreased in the skin and lungs, thus accounting for the increased toxicity seen in these organs with systemic exposure. However, when given intradermally, bleomycin is concentrated at the site of injection where it is slowly inactivated while systemic levels and systemic side effects are minimized.[10]

CLINICAL EVIDENCE

Several studies have examined the efficacy of intralesional bleomycin in the treatment of warts (Table 10.1). Shumer and O'Keefe[11] performed a double-masked, placebo-controlled, crossover study on recalcitrant

warts in 40 patients. Patients were alternately assigned to one of two groups and injected with up to 1 ml of bleomycin 1 U/ml or physiological (0.9%) saline. Injections occurred at 2-week intervals. Of the warts, 60% of plantar warts, 94% of periungual warts and 95% of warts at other sites were cured after one or two injections, for an overall success rate of 81%. None of the warts injected with saline responded.

In a similar study by Bunney et al,[12] 59 matched pairs of recalcitrant hand warts were blindly treated with up to 0.2 ml of either bleomycin 1 U/ml or 0.9% saline at 3-week intervals. At 6 weeks, they found 87.5% of patients responded favorably to bleomycin with 58% cured. Only 10% of those treated with 0.9% saline were cured. At 12 weeks (four treatments), 76% of warts treated with bleomycin were cured. In a parallel study of patients with resistant warts, 75% of hand warts were cured and 66% of mosaic plantar warts were cured.

In a randomized double-blind study, Hayes and O'Keefe[13] showed that a reduced dose of bleomycin was equally effective in the treatment of recalcitrant warts. Warts were injected with bleomycin at concentrations of 0.25 U/ml, 0.5 U/ml or 1 U/ml. The volume injected varied according to the size of the wart. Warts up to 5 mm received 0.2 ml, those up to 10 mm received 0.2–0.5 ml and larger warts received up to 1.0 ml. Treatment with bleomycin 0.5 U/ml was found to be as effective as 1 U/ml. Although bleomycin 0.25 U/ml cured 73.3% of warts, not enough warts were treated to make a statistically significant conclusion about this lower concentration. Overall, 78% of the 79 warts treated with bleomycin resolved after one to three injections at 3-week intervals.

Several non-blinded placebo-controlled studies have demonstrated similar results with bleomycin. Amer et al[14] injected up to 0.2 ml of bleomycin 1 U/ml into 143 warts and saline into 35 paired warts in the same patients. They

Table 10.1 Clinical study outcomes

Reference	Dose of bleomycin per injection (U/ml)	Number of injections	Percentage resolved with bleomycin	Percentage resolved with placebo
Shumer and O'Keefe[11]	1 up to 1 ml	1–2	81	0
Bunney et al[12]	1 up to 0.2 ml	1–3	76	10
Hayes and O'Keefe[13]	0.5, 1 up to 1 ml	1–3	86, 73	N/A
Amer et al[14]	1 up to 0.2 ml	1–2	67.8	2.9
Shumack and Haddock[15]	1	1–3	99.23	0
Cordero et al[17]	1 up to 0.8 ml	1–2	75	N/A
Bremner[16]	1 up to 1 ml	1–2	63	N/A
Abbott[18]	1 up to 0.2 ml	1–> 6	50[a]	N/A
Hudson[2]	1 up to 1 ml	1–3	100	N/A
Munkvad et al[1]	1 up to 0.4 ml	3	18–23	45

[a]Given as percentage of patients cleared, not as percentage of warts cleared.

achieved a 67.8% cure rate in the bleomycin-treated warts as opposed to a 2.9% cure rate in the saline group. Shumack and Haddock[15] achieved a 99.23% cure rate at 12 weeks after injecting 1052 warts with bleomycin 1 U/ml. In the study, 40 warts injected with saline showed no signs of regression at 6 weeks. After these same warts were reinjected with bleomycin (crossover design), all 40 warts resolved.

Many uncontrolled studies have reported comparable benefits in the treatment of warts with bleomycin. Hudson[2] reports resolution in 22 of 25 patients with refractory plantar warts after one injection of up to 1 ml bleomycin 1 U/ml. The three remaining patients cleared after two or three injections. Bremner et al[16] treated 142 warts in 24 patients with up to 1 ml of bleomycin 1 U/ml and reported a 63% cure rate. Cordero et al[17] treated 36 patients with up to 0.8 ml of bleomycin 1 U/ml and achieved cure rates of 67% in plantar warts, 82% in periungual warts and 80% in other warts. Abbott[18] used 0.2 ml of bleomycin 1 U/ml in multiple injections and achieved a patient cure rate of almost 50%.

Opposing the previously mentioned clinical research, two studies found bleomycin to be no better than placebo in double-blinded trials. Munkvad et al[1] treated 108 warts on 62 patients with one of four injectables: bleomycin 1 U/ml up to 0.4 ml in saline or oil, 0.9% saline or sesame oil.[1] The cure rates were 18% and 23% with bleomycin in saline and oil, respectively. Interestingly, the combined placebo groups showed a cure rate of 45%. This was a statistically significant difference from the combined active groups. However, this study is thought to be flawed because the authors did not ensure that the groups were similar with respect to size and location of warts.[10] They also never explained how they pooled their data or stated the significance level.[10] Perez et al[19] also found that the injection of bleomycin into warts is not statistically better than the injection of saline (see Evidence-based Medicine rating, page 13).

The Cochrane database of reviews in 2000 used five randomized controlled trials to conclude that there is 'insufficient evidence of efficacy' to warrant the use of bleomycin.[31] However, Sterling et al[27] in 2001 found the treat-

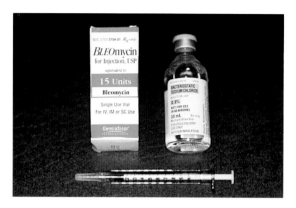

Figure 10.1
Box and vial of bleomycin along with syringe needed for injection.

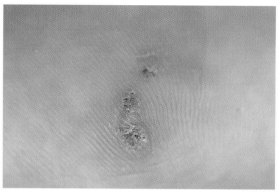

Figure 10.2
Wart on the foot 1 week after treatment with bleomycin.

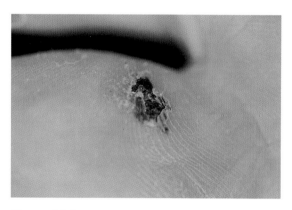

Figure 10.3
Plantar wart on the great toe 2 weeks after treatment with bleomycin.

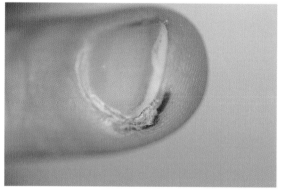

Figure 10.4
Warts on the middle finger 2 weeks after treatment with bleomycin.

ment of warts with bleomycin to be level BIIii based on strength of evidence. This suggests that there is 'fair evidence to support the use of the procedure'. We feel more strongly about the evidence. There are at least four randomized controlled clinical trials supporting the use of bleomycin, and multiple case series that also provide evidence of its effectiveness. The two studies that did not show efficacy appear to have been flawed and, therefore, the evidence

is largely homogenous. Using our Modified Evidence-based Medicine system, the strength of evidence for using bleomycin for the treatment of warts is rated level 1 (see Chapter 19).

CASE REPORT

A 28-year-old woman was referred to the dermatology clinic for a 3-year history of a

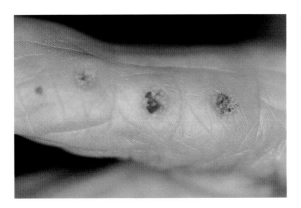

Figure 10.5
Warts on the index finger 2 weeks after
treatment with bleomycin.

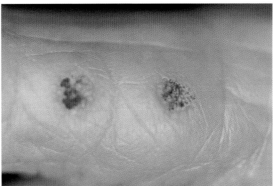

Figure 10.6
Close-up picture of the wart in Figure 10.5.

**Table 10.2 Favored treatment
methodology**

1. Bleomycin sulfate can be prepared by
   mixing the 15-unit vial of bleomycin with
   30 ml 0.9% sodium chloride formulated
   for injection. This will provide 0.5 U/ml of
   bleomycin sulfate
2. The wart should not be pared before the
   initial treatment
3. After cleansing the wart with isopropyl
   alcohol, inject the bleomycin sulfate into
   the base of the wart parallel to the skin.
   Perfuse the wart to allow maximum
   exposure to the bleomycin. A 1-ml
   Luerlock syringe with a 30-gauge needle
   should be used. Avoid injecting
   subcutaneously, as this will increase pain
   and decrease effectiveness
4. Pain can be expected during the next 72
   hours, but often less than with
   cryosurgery. A hemorrhagic blister may
   occur. No drainage is necessary unless
   pain is severe. The hemorrhagic blister is
   usually a good prognostic indicator
5. The wart should be evaluated at 3- to 4-
   week intervals with re-treatment of
   persistent wart after paring

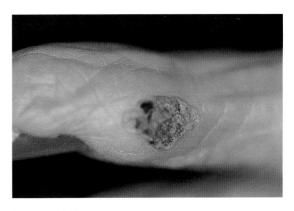

Figure 10.7
Wart on the finger 2 weeks after treatment
with bleomycin.

2.6-mm wart on the middle phalanx of her right
little finger.[10] She had used several over-the-
counter topical salicylic acid products for years
and cryotherapy was used on four occasions,
but the wart recurred. After obtaining informed
consent she was given 0.5 ml of a 0.5 U/ml
intralesional injection of bleomycin sulfate.
Four weeks later, residual wart was still apparent and a second injection was given. One

month later the wart had completely resolved. The patient remains lesion-free 16 months later with no evidence of scarring.

FAVORED TREATMENT METHODOLOGY (Table 10.2)

Bleomycin is commonly used for warts that have failed to respond to other treatment approaches. We recommend that bleomycin be used as a third-line treatment for warts (Figures 10.1–10.7). Studies have used concentrations of bleomycin of 0.25–1 U/ml with no advantages for higher doses. To reduce discomfort, bleomycin should be reconstituted in 1% lignocaine (lidocaine).[20] There have been a variety of methods used to inject bleomycin into warts. Some of these methods include direct intralesional injection with a needle and syringe, 'pricking' with a Monolet needle, 'bleopuncture', pressure-sensitive tape containing bleomycin and a modified tattooing machine known as dermatography.[20 24] Optimal results are obtained when the intralesional injection produces a blanching of the wart. This can be accomplished by injecting the base of the wart parallel to the skin, which allows maximum perfusion of the wart. Subcutaneous injection should be avoided. A haemorrhagic blister may occur within 2–3 days. The eschar should be pared after 3–4 weeks. Additional treatments should be repeated at 3- to 4-week intervals until cure has been obtained. Bleomycin will remain active for 3 months if stored at 4°C.[13]

ADVERSE EFFECTS

Intralesional bleomycin injection is very well tolerated and there have been relatively few side effects reported. The most common adverse effect is pain during and after the injection. By 48 hours the pain typically subsides.

Raynaud's phenomenon has been reported in several cases of bleomycin injection. If it proves to be common, this debilitating problem would limit its use.[25] Most cases have occurred after injection into a digit, although Vanhooteghem et al[26] report one case of Raynaud's phenomenon occurring after injection into the sole.

Other uncommon effects of bleomycin include edema, hematoma, scarring, pigmentary changes, local urticaria and nail damage.[13,27,28] Urbina et al[29] reported a case in which a 15-year-old completely lost two fingernails after two periungual injections of 0.15 U bleomycin. There were no signs of regrowth at

Table 10.3 Patient education sheet

What is bleomycin?
Bleomycin is a powerful medication used to treat both benign and malignant tumors. Bleomycin is injected locally into warts and helps kill the virus-infected cells.

What are the side effects?
The most common side effect of bleomycin treatment is pain at the injection site. An eschar (black crust) at the treatment site is expected a few days after treatment. Other uncommon effects include swelling, nail damage and skin color change. Raynaud's phenomenon is a condition where fingers or toes change color and become painful when exposed to cold temperatures. This is a rare but serious adverse effect associated with bleomycin injection into fingers and toes. Re-treatment may be needed.

How long will it take to work?
Within a few days after the injection, a dark scab will form and surrounding skin may turn pink. The scab (and wart) will eventually fall off or can be pared away. A repeat injection may be required if the wart persists beyond 4 weeks.

a 6-month follow-up. Allen and Fusko[30] reported a case of cellulitis and bacterial lymphangitis after treatment of a plantar wart. (The patient was treated with antibiotics and improved without sequelae, although the patient's wart never resolved.)

Systemic toxicity is rarely reported even though plasma levels may be as high as 113.5 ng/ml when 1 ml of bleomycin 1 U/ml is injected.[9] Bleomycin has been shown to be teratogenic in mice, so pregnant patients should not be treated.[26] No studies on the long-term effects of bleomycin have been conducted.

COURSE AND PROGNOSIS

The injection of bleomycin causes some pain, but this should not persist beyond 72 hours. A hemorrhagic necrotic eschar is expected to occur about 2–3 days after treatment. This will eventually fall off or can be pared away. Bleomycin injection typically produces little, if any, scarring and other side effects are rare. Success rates vary, as noted in the clinical evidence section. A patient examination sheet (Table 10.3) is helpful.

REFERENCES

1. Munkvad M, Genner J, Staberg B, Kongsholm H. Locally injected bleomycin in the treatment of warts. *Dermatologica* 1983; **167**: 86–9.
2. Hudson AL. Letter: Treatment of plantar warts with bleomycin. *Arch Dermatol* 1976; **112**: 1179.
3. Umezaqa H, Maeda K, Takeuchi T, Okami Y. New antibiotics, bleomycin A and B. *J Antibiot* 1966; **19**: 200.
4. Suzuki Y, Miyake H, Sakai M, Inuyama Y, Matsukawa J, Fujii K. Bleomycin in malignant tumors of head and neck. *Keio J Med* 1969; **18**: 153–62.

5. Gilman AG, Hardman JG, Limbird LE. In: *Goodman and Gilman's The Pharmacological Basis of Therapeutics*, 10th edn. McGraw-Hill, New York, 2001: 1429–40.
6. In: Katzung BG. *Basic and Clinical Pharmacology*, 8th edn. Lang Medical Books/ McGraw-Hill, New York, 2001: 940.
7. Templeton SF, Solomon AR, Swerlick RA. Intra-dermal bleomycin injections into normal human skin. A histopathologic and immunopathologic study. *Arch Dermatol* 1994; **130**: 577–83.
8. Sobh MA, Abd El-Razic MM, Rizc RA, Eid MM, Abd el-Hamid IA, Ghoneim MA. Intralesional injection of bleomycin sulphate into resistant warts in renal transplant recipients versus non-transplant warty patients. *Acta Dermato-Venereol* 1991; **71**: 63–6.
9. James MP, Collier PM, Aherne W, Hardcastle A, Lovegrove S. Histologic, pharmacologic, and immunocytochemical effects of injection of bleomycin into viral warts. *J Am Acad Dermatol* 1993; **28**: 933–7.
10. Chan S, Middleton RK. Bleomycin treatment of warts. *Drug Intell Clin Pharm* 1990; **24**: 952–3.
11. Shumer SM, O'Keefe EJ. Bleomycin in the treatment of recalcitrant warts. *J Am Acad Dermatol* 1983; **9**: 91–6.
12. Bunney MH, Nolan MW, Buxton PK, Going SM, Prescott RJ. The treatment of resistant warts with intralesional bleomycin: a controlled clinical trial. *Br J Dermatol* 1984; **111**: 197–207.
13. Hayes ME, O'Keefe EJ. Reduced dose of bleomycin in the treatment of recalcitrant warts. *J Am Acad Dermatol* 1986; **15**(5 Pt1): 1002–6.
14. Amer M, Diab N, Ramadan A, Galal A, Salem A. Therapeutic evaluation for intralesional injection of bleomycin sulfate in 143 resistant warts. *J Am Acad Dermatol* 1988; **18**: 1313–16.
15. Shumack PH, Haddock MJ. Bleomycin: an effective treatment for warts. *Austral J Dermatol* 1979; **20**: 41–2.
16. Bremner RM. Warts: treatment with intralesional bleomycin. *Cutis* 1976; **18**: 264–6.

17. Cordero AA, Guglielmi HA, Woscoff A. The common wart: intralesional treatment with bleomycin sulfate. *Cutis* 1980; **26**: 319–20, 322, 324.

18. Abbott LG. Treatment of warts with bleomycin. *Austral J Dermatol* 1978; **19**: 69–71.

19. Perez A, Weiss E, Piquero MJ. Hypertronic saline solution vs intralesional bleomycin in the treatment of common warts. *Dermatol Venez* 1992; **30**: 176–8.

20. Manz LA, Pelachyk JM. Bleomycin–lidocaine mixture reduces pain of intralesional injection in the treatment of recalcitrant verrucae. *J Am Acad Dermatol* 1991; **25**: 524–6.

21. Munn SE, Higgins E, Marshall M, Clement M. A new method of intralesional bleomycin therapy in the treatment of recalcitrant warts. *Br J Dermatol* 1996; **135**: 969–71.

22. Shelley WB, Shelley ED. Intralesional bleomycin sulfate therapy for warts. A novel bifurcated needle puncture technique. *Arch Dermatol* 1991; **127**: 234–6.

23. Takigawa M, Oku T, Ginoza M, Yamada M, Yamamoto T, Kobayashi I. Treatment of viral warts with pressure-sensitive adhesive tape containing bleomycin sulfate. *Arch Dermatol* 1985; **121**: 1108.

24. van der Velden EM, Ijsselmuiden OE, Drost BH, Baruchin AM. Dermatography with bleomycin as a new treatment for verrucae vulgaris. *Int J Dermatol* 1997; **36**: 145–50.

25. Epstein E. Intralesional bleomycin and Raynaud's phenomenon. *J Am Acad Dermatol* 1991; **24**(5 Pt 1): 785–6.

26. Vanhooteghem O, Richert B, de la Brassinne M. Raynaud phenomenon after treatment of verruca vulgaris of the sole with intralesional injection of bleomycin. *Pediatr Dermatol* 2001; **18**: 449–51.

27. Sterling JC, Handfield-Jones S, Hudson PM. Guidelines for the management of cutaneous warts. *Br J Dermatol* 2001; **144**: 4–11.

28. Miller RA. Nail dystrophy following intralesional injections of bleomycin for a periungual wart. *Arch Dermatol* 1984; **120**: 963–4.

29. Urbina Gonzalez F, Cristobal Gil MC, Aguilar Martinez A, Guerra Rodriguez P, Sanchez de Paz E, Garcia-Perez A. Cutaneous toxicity of intralesional bleomycin administration in the treatment of periungual warts. *Arch Dermatol* 1986; **122**: 974–5.

30. Allen AL, Fosko SW. Lymphangitis as a complication of intralesional bleomycin therapy. *J Am Acad Dermatol* 1998; **39** (2 Pt 1): 295–7.

31. Gibbs S, Harvey I, Sterling JC, Stark R. Local treatments for cutaneous warts. *The Cochrane Database of Systematic Reviews* Vol 3, 2001.

11 Laser therapy

Geeta Mohla Shah and Stephen E Helms

Historical aspects • Carbon dioxide laser • Pulsed dye laser • Conclusion • References

Laser is an acronym for light amplification by stimulated emission of radiation. Lasers generate an intense beam of light energy in the form of photons that are synchronized in time and space, and usually share the same wavelength. The wavelength of the beam is formed when specific atoms are stimulated with either a light, radiofrequency, electrical, or chemical energy source. When these atoms return spontaneously to their stable state, they give off photons of energy with a wavelength specific to the excited molecule. This process is amplified by the use of reflective mirrors in a 'laser tube' or 'resonating chamber'. The laser beam escapes the chamber when the energy of the stimulated amplified emission of photons reaches a certain threshold.[1,2]

Lasers have been used in dermatology for many different conditions ranging from vascular lesions, benign and malignant growths, to epidermal resurfacing. Several lasers have been used to treat warts, including the carbon dioxide laser, pulsed-dye laser, alexandrite laser, and erbium–YAG (yttrium–aluminum–garnet) laser. The carbon dioxide and flashlamp pulsed dye lasers have been used most in the treatment of warts and are the focus of this chapter.

HISTORICAL ASPECTS

The fundamental basis of lasers was established in the early 1900s with Albert Einstein's theory of stimulated emission of photons. In 1959, the first laser was developed by Theodore Maiman; however, it was not until 1963 that the first cutaneous applications of lasers were introduced by Dr Leon Goldman, a dermatologist. The carbon dioxide (CO_2) laser was developed by Patel and colleagues in 1964.[1,3,4] Over time, more sophisticated lasers have been developed that target specific components of skin. In the 1980s, Anderson and Parrish[5] elucidated the principles of selective photothermolysis, in which they described how controlled destruction of targeted lesional tissue was possible with minimal thermal damage to surrounding tissues.

CARBON DIOXIDE LASER

Basic science

The emission wavelength of the CO_2 laser is 10 600 nm, i.e. in the far infrared part of the electromagnetic spectrum. This corresponds to the absorption band of water. In treated tissue, the laser beam targets intracellular water and causes a release of heat that irreversibly vaporizes tissue proteins, with little dissipation in the adjacent skin. This allows for controlled vaporization of tissue. In fact, the thermal damage to the target and surrounding tissue is proportional to the duration of exposure. An added benefit of the CO_2 laser tissue ablation is to provide hemostasis, allowing for a relatively bloodless field during treatment.[2,6]

Energy is the capacity to do work. The unit of measurement of energy is the joule (J), which is 1 watt (W) × 1 second (s). The dosage of energy delivered by a laser to tissue is described in specific terms. The power density or irradiance is the rate of energy delivered per unit of target tissue area. It is expressed as watts per square centimeter (W/cm^2). This is determined by the power of the laser divided by the surface area of the beam, which is usually termed 'the spot size'. The area of a circle varies as the square of its radius and, therefore, a reduction in spot size by one half would produce a fourfold increase in the power density. Another method of altering energy delivered to tissue involves moving the hand piece of the laser apparatus farther from the target tissue than the focused beam, controlled by a fixed guide on the laser hand piece. The defocused beam will provide less energy. The power density, however, does not account for time. Fluence is the total energy impacting the tissue over time. This is expressed as joules per square centimeter (J/cm^2). Fluence can be calculated from the power density (irradiance) and the exposure time. The final factor controlled by the laser operator is the pulse duration.[6] The CO_2 laser on a continuous mode emits a beam of light, as long as the foot pedal is depressed. CO_2 laser light can also be delivered in pulses of varying lengths and at intervals of varying frequency, including the new superpulsed and ultrapulsed lasers that emit a controlled train of short-duration high-power pulses.

Clinical evidence

The CO_2 laser is useful for vaporization of various epidermal and dermal lesions (Figure 11.1). Common indications for the CO_2 laser

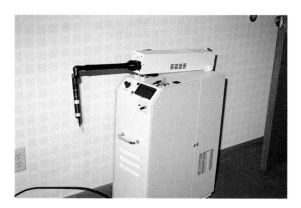

Figure 11.1
A CO_2 laser with an articulated hand piece.

include photo-induced facial wrinkles, actinic cheilitis, atrophic scars, and rhinophyma.[4] The CO_2 laser has also been used to treat condyloma acuminatum, periungual verrucae, and palmar/plantar verrucae. No randomized controlled, masked trials are present in the dermatology literature regarding CO_2 laser treatment of warts. In fact, such studies would be almost impossible to design because the patient and researcher would observe the defect created by the vaporization of the wart in the treatment group. Many case series have shown this laser to be an effective treatment modality when more traditional methods have failed. It has also been used as initial therapy in selected cases. An early study in 1980 demonstrated a very impressive 94.7% success rate in 75 plantar warts treated only once with the CO_2 laser.[7] However, other studies reported significantly lower cure rates of 32–64.1%.[8–10] Some studies showed lower rates for recalcitrant lesions with better rates for primary treatments[11] and others had intermediate results[12,13] (Table 11.1). It is unclear why the cure rates vary to such a great extent. Certainly the results are operator dependent, and furthermore the size, location, number, and duration of the warts as well as previous therapy may be important determinants of

Table 11.1 CO_2 laser treatment of verrucae

Authors	Number treated	Site	Previously treated	Results
Mueller et al[6]	75	Plantar	Yes	94.7% success rate after one treatment
McBurney and Rosen[11]	27	Periungual and plantar	Yes	81% clear after one treatment, 15% clear after two treatments, 4% clear after three treatments
Logan and Zachary[7]	18	Plantar, periungual, and fingers/hands	Yes	Overall cure rate of 56%
Apfelberg et al[8]	25	Periungual, subungual, and mosaic	Yes	32% with permanent cure, 52% with complete or partial cure
Street and Roenigk[12]	24	Periungual	Yes	71% clearing with one to two treatments
Lim and Goh[10]	68	Periungual and subungual	40 had failed previous treatments, 20 were treated with CO_2 laser as first-line treatment	Recalcitrant verrucae had a cure rate of 48% whereas first-time treatment lesions had a cure rate of 80%
Sloan K et al[9]	200	Plantar, periungual and other verrucae (on hands, face, torso)	Yes	Overall cure of 64.1% after one treatment. 71% were satisfied with results

success, although analysis of these factors has not always shown statistical significance.[10] The CO_2 laser can also be used to treat external genital warts. Cure rates of over 90% have been reported in patients with external genital and perianal condyloma acuminata after only one treatment with the CO_2 laser.[14] Bar-Am et al.[15] studied 119 men with recalcitrant genital condylomata; 82% of these patients were cured after just one treatment, with the remainder achieving cure by the end of the third treatment. Using our Modified Evidence-based Medicine system (Chapter 19) we classify CO_2 laser therapy of warts as level III

evidence. Though there is some homogeneity of cohort studies, the wide range of cure rates is of concern.

Favored treatment methodology

Patient education is very important because laser concepts are not well understood by most patients (Table 11.2). When treating plantar warts, a 2- to 3-mm margin is drawn

Table 11.2 Patient education sheet CO$_2$ laser

General information

Laser is an acronym for <u>l</u>ight <u>a</u>mplification by <u>s</u>timulated <u>e</u>mission of <u>r</u>adiation. This means that lasers generate an intense beam of light energy. When this light is absorbed by the water in your skin, tremendous heat is generated. The skin actually boils and bubbling can be seen. The amount of heating is controlled by the doctor. This requires a local anesthetic and small injections are given under the skin surrounding the warts that will be treated. You will also be required to wear glasses or goggles when the laser is operational.

Day of treatment

- Clean warts with soap and water the morning of your treatment
- Tell your doctor if you have any medicine allergies or seizure disorder
- Wear comfortable clothing that can be easily removed to expose the area to be treated
- You will see bright flashes of light during the treatment
- Let your doctor know if you feel any pain during the treatment

Post-treatment instructions

- Apply antibiotic ointment twice daily to the treatment site
- Cover with a non-stick dressing
- Call your doctor if you have increasing pain, yellow drainage, expanding redness, a red streak, fever, or any other unusual symptoms

around the wart and local anesthesia is administered using 1% lidocaine with epinephrine. A regional posterior tibial nerve block, using 1% lidocaine without epinephrine, may be used along with local infiltration. A continuous wave-defocused CO$_2$ laser should be used at 15–20 W power output. The visible wart tissue, along with the margin, should be vaporized, painting the surface of the wart by a slow continuous motion until the surface is charred. The char should be removed with a wet gauze and then wiped with a dry gauze. The process is repeated, vaporizing another layer of the wart, and more char is removed. It should be noted that wart tissue produces a bubbly appearance when being vaporized. Normal dermis beneath the lesion appears to melt. Furthermore, warts interrupt the dermatoglyphic lines of the skin. When the wart is completely vaporized, these dermatoglyphic lines pass through the treated area. A smoke evacuator should be used during the vaporization process. Postoperatively, the treated area appears white and may develop localized swelling. In the following few days, the area will appear erythematous, and granulation tissue develops 5–10 days postoperatively. The treated area heals in 2–12 weeks. Postoperative care should include cleaning the wound with tap water once or twice a day. Wound care with antibiotic ointments under non-stick pads (Telfa) is used to provide the best healing environment, and to speed re-epithelialization and decrease scarring and pain. The treated area should be elevated when possible during the first few days to decrease swelling. We use acetaminophen (paracetamol) or propoxyphene/acetaminophen as needed for pain. The CO$_2$ laser should be used cautiously, and only after the risks and benefits have been discussed, with patients who have diabetes mellitus, peripheral vascular disease, peripheral neuropathy, or a history of poor wound healing.

For treatment of periungual warts, a 2- to 4-mm margin should be drawn around the wart. A digital nerve block may be used with additional local anesthesia if necessary. Complete or partial nail avulsion may be performed with the laser when subungual wart is present. The wart is vaporized with a series of passes using the process described above. Wound care should be directed as above.

When treating condylomata acuminata, 2- to 3-mm margins should be used because of the risk of malignancy in these areas. The area should be anesthetized with 1% lidocaine and normal tissue should be covered with wet gauze. Thin condylomata can usually be vaporized intact; however, thicker papillomatous lesions may be excised first with the continuous CO^2 laser with a focused beam at 15–20 W of power output, followed by vaporization of the base with a defocused beam at 10–15 W of power output. The treated area should be wiped with a wet gauze and then dried. This process should be repeated until bubbling ceases and a smooth, whitened mucosa is seen, signaling the endpoint of treatment. The treated areas should be cleaned with soap and water followed by application of antibiotic solution and a non-adherent dressing. The area often takes 4–6 weeks to heal.[16]

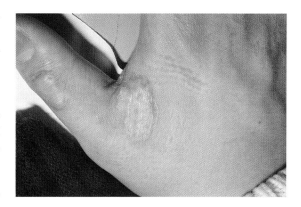

Figure 11.2
Hypertrophic scarring 1 month after CO_2 laser vaporization of two warts on the dorsum of the right hand and thumb. The patient used the same Telfa dressings over bacitractin/polymyxin B ointment used by other patients discussed elsewhere, and did not report any local infection during the healing process.

Adverse effects and laser safety

Side effects may occur in 1–4% of cases after CO_2 laser treatment,[16] but have been reported in as many as 61%.[8] These adverse effects include scarring, pain, and prolonged healing. Scarring may be hypertrophic or atrophic, with atrophic scarring occurring more often on the hands (Figure 11.2). Logan and Zachary[8] reported scarring in 61% of the patients in

their study. Nail changes may occur after treatment of periungual and subungual warts, and include distal onycholysis, nail thickening, nail curvature, and grooves.[13] These changes are usually temporary. Numbness and pain have also been reported. Pain is usually reported as minimal; however, in one study, two patients had significant pain with decreased function.[13] While performing the procedure, burns may occur on the patient, operating room personnel, or surgeon's hands.

In addition, viable human papillomavirus (HPV) DNA has been identified in the CO_2 laser plume and preventive measures such as facemasks and smoke evacuators are essential.[18] Similarly, laser treatment may be accompanied by a noxious odor and the release of a 'lung-damaging dust' that can penetrate the deepest portion of the lungs. The risks of inhaling this smoke are unknown.[17] The vacuum-powered smoke evacuator should be placed 1 cm away from the laser plume. The smoke evacuator is 98.6% efficient at removing viral particles when placed 1 cm away from the treatment site, but its efficiency drops to 50% when placed 2 cm away.[19] Although reports of HPV infection acquired through the laser plume have not been made with the pulsed dye or

CO_2 lasers for common warts, precautions should still be taken as a result of a report of laryngeal papillomatosis in a surgeon who was treating anogenital condylomata.[20] A patient education handout that emphasizes possible side effects is often useful (see Table 11.2).

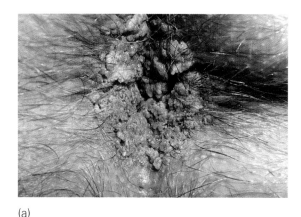

(a)

Figure 11.3
(a) A large expanding mass of perianal warts is present. There was little improvement with liquid nitrogen cryotherapy, podophyllin home therapy, and imiquimod home therapy. (b) This is the appearance of the perianal skin immediately after ablation of the wart with CO_2 laser. (c) One week after CO_2 laser ablation and treatment with bacitractin/polymyxin B ointment four times a day, the wound is moist and re-epithelialization is present in many areas. (d) Complete re-epithelialization has occurred 3 weeks after CO_2 laser ablation, with white pinpoint areas representing centers of re-epithelialization centered on hair follicles. No recurrent wart is present.

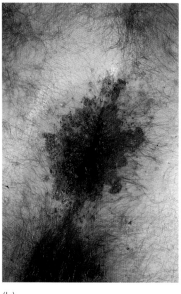

(b)

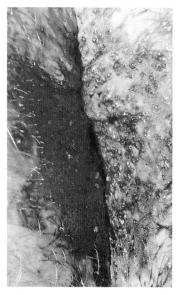

(c)

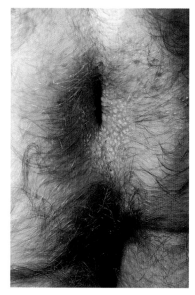

(d)

Cost–benefit considerations

The cost of any treatment is always important but cost-effectiveness is the proper way to understand the true cost of any modality. Two studies that looked at CO_2 laser therapy of condylomata acuminata found laser treatment to be cost-effective when compared with other surgical procedures or physician-administered medical therapies.[21,22]

Reimbursement for CO_2 laser therapy for warts in the USA is based on CPT codes. Wart treatment payments are identical for destruction by any method including chemical, cryosurgical, or electrical fulguration. These payments are relatively low and do not account for the $US30 000–40 000 expense of purchasing a CO_2 laser or the training required for its optimal use. The numbers of patients treated monthly with this modality, as well as the reimbursement by the prevailing healthcare system(s), are needed to determine the economic viability of this technology. As a result of its cost, laser therapy is generally not instituted as first-line treatment of warts and is most often used when other modalities have failed. For resistant warts unresponsive to other modalities, the CO_2 laser may be a logical alternative.

Case reports

Case 1

A 35-year-old heterosexual man presented for evaluation of perianal warts, which had increased in number and size over the past 2 years (Figure 11.3a). The lesions were tender, bled intermittently, and were difficult to keep clean after bowel movements. He had previously been treated with liquid nitrogen cryotherapy on five occasions, followed by a course of home therapy with podofilox 0.5% gel (Condylox™, *Dak Pharmaceuticals,*

Philadelphia, PA, USA) twice daily for 3 days each week for 2 months, and then 0.5% imiquimod cream applied at bedtime, on Monday, Wednesday, and Friday for 8 weeks, with no sustained improvement. After discussing the risks and benefits of CO_2 laser surgery, the area was cleansed with hydrogen peroxide and anesthetized using 1% lidocaine with epinephrine. With a power density of 20 W/cm^2 the CO_2 laser was used to 'paint' over the lesion with a slow, steady motion using the continuous mode, until the surface was uniformly charred. The black char was wiped away with a moist gauze, and eight additional passes of the CO_2 laser led to resolution of all visible wart (Figure 11.3b). The patient was instructed to apply bacitracin/polymyxin ointment (Polysporin™, *Pfizer Inc., Terre Haute, IN, USA*) four times a day to the wound, and to eat bran with each meal to soften his stool. He also took ketorolac trometamol (Toradol) 10 mg every 6 hours as needed for pain. One week later the wound showed moist, bright-red granulation tissue and was partially re-epithelialized (Figure 11.3c). Three weeks after CO_2 laser ablation, the treated area had completely re-epithelialized (Figure 11.3d). Anoscopy at this time revealed no internal warts. One year later the patient remained free of recurrence.

Case 2

A 24-year-old presented with a confluent mosaic wart over the plantar surface of the right big toe. Wart was also present on the right second toe in a 10 × 6 mm area, including the skin where the second toe touches the big toe. The patient had used salicylic acid daily for 1 year and showed only transient thinning of the wart after each of three treatments with liquid nitrogen cryotherapy. After discussing risks and benefits, the wart was treated with the CO_2 laser after a digital block was

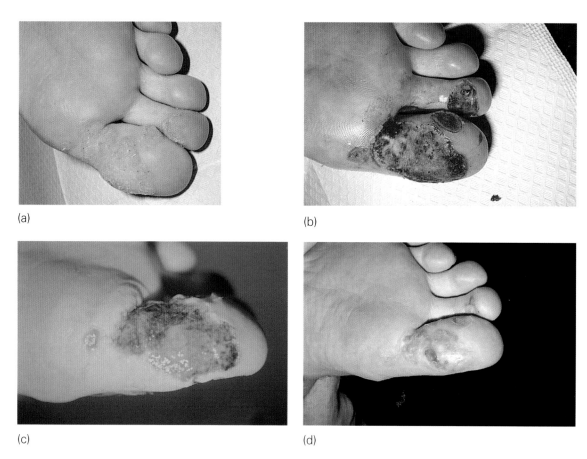

(a)

(b)

(c)

(d)

Figure 11.4
(a) Confluent growth in a large mosaic wart is present over the plantar surface of the right big toe, right second toe, and the ball of the foot. Numerous thrombosed capillaries are noted. (b) Immediately after CO_2 laser ablation, the dermatoglyphic markings are still visible in the dermis. (c) One week after CO_2 laser ablation, moist granulation tissue is present over the wound, which has been treated with Telfa dressings over bacitracin/polymyxin B ointment. (d) Four weeks after CO_2 laser vaporization, the completely healed wound blistered following a 2-mile run (3 km), leaving the shallow erosion noted at the center. Using a Band-Aid™ (*Johnson & Johnson, New Brunswick, NJ, USA*) prior to jogging prevented further friction blistering.

performed on the right big toe and second toe using 1% lidocaine without epinephrine. Additional local injections of 1% lidocaine were used proximally on the big toe. With a power density of 20 W/cm^2 and a continuous laser mode, the area was painted with a slow steady motion until the entire wart was charred. After each of six passes, the char was wiped away with a gauze soaked in tap water. At the time the tissue no longer 'bubbled' in response to the laser and dermatoglyphs were visible through the entire area, suggesting that the lesion had been entirely ablated (Figure 11.4b). Bacitracin/polymyxin ointment (Polysporin) was applied under a non-stick pad (Telfa) with daily cleaning with tap water. One week later, the wound showed excellent red moist granulation tissue (Figure 11.4c). Four weeks after CO_2 laser surgery, the wound was completely healed, but a small blister had developed within the healed area from friction while jogging the day before. The patient applied a Band-Aid before jogging for the next 6 months and further blisters did not occur. One year later, the patient returned with a 1-mm diameter wart on the right big toe adjacent to the area treated by laser. This was treated with liquid nitrogen cryotherapy for 25 seconds followed by daily salicylic acid home treatments, and the wart did not recur.

PULSED DYE LASER

Basic science

The flashlamp pulsed dye laser (PDL) emits a yellow light with a wavelength of 585, 595, or 600 nm, which can selectively target oxyhemoglobin in blood vessels. The idea of treating warts with this laser is rooted in the concept of selective photothermolysis. In the 1980s, Anderson and Parrish[5] elucidated the principles of selective photothermolysis in which they described how controlled destruction of targeted lesional tissue was possible with minimal thermal damage to surrounding tissues. In this theory, a targeted tissue (chromophore) can be selectively damaged with a light pulse that is of a certain wavelength and has a shorter pulse duration than the thermal relaxation time of the chromophore. The targeted chromophore dissipates the heat to its surroundings through thermal diffusion. The specified time for an object to lose heat energy to the surrounding tissue is the thermal relaxation time. This is defined as the time required for the targeted site to cool to one-half of its peak temperature immediately after laser irradiation.[4,23] The use of laser pulses that are shorter than the thermal relaxation time of a chromophore does not allow enough time for heat to diffuse to adjacent tissue, thus confining damage to the target and limiting collateral injury.[23]

Dilated blood vessels within the wart are 'cauterized' as the targeted hemoglobin is heated. As blood flow to the wart is compromised, all or a portion of the wart becomes necrotic and sloughs. As the blood vessels are selectively targeted, minimal damage occurs to the surrounding tissue.[24] Tan et al[24] examined the histological changes that occur after wart treatment with the PDL. Immediately after therapy, coagulated red cells were visualized in the papillary vessels; 24 hours later, necrosis and vacuolization of the keratinocytes and blood vessel walls were noted. These changes persisted at 6–13 days after treatment.[24] By specifying wavelength (585 or 595 nm), pulse duration (1.5 ms), and fluence (10–20 J/cm^2), laser parameters can be customized for treatment of warts, allowing for maximal destruction of blood vessels within a wart but minimizing damage to adjoining structures.[4]

Clinical evidence

Early studies with the 585-nm flashlamp PDL established remarkable effectiveness in treating verrucae. Tan et al[24] performed an open study using PDL treatment of 39 patients with recalcitrant warts. In this study, warts were pared before treatment and single 5-mm spotsize pulses were delivered to each wart. Of all of the treated warts, 72% cleared after an average of 1.68 treatments. Periungual verrucae had a clearance rate of 85.7% after 1.85 treatments, whereas 83% of warts on other areas responded after 1.4 treatments. Plantar warts had the poorest response rate of 50%. A recurrence rate of 3.6% was noted during the 5-month follow-up period.[24]

Table 11.3 Comparison of studies of pulsed dye laser (PDL) therapy for verrucae

Authors	No. of warts	Wart type	Wart location	Pared before treatment	Fluence (J/cm^2)	Average no. of treatments	Clearance rate (%)	Recurrence rate (%)
Tan et al[25]	39	Recal	All sites	Yes	6.25–7.5	1.68	72	3.6
Kauvar et al[6]	728	703 Recal 25 no previous tx	All sites	Yes	7.0–9.5	2.5	93	
Webster et al[27]	54	Recal	All sites	No	6.75–10	2.5	52	
Borovoy et al[31]	200	194 Recal 6 no previous tx	Plantar	Yes	6.5–9	2.38	80	0
Jain et al[32]	97		Plantar	Yes	8.1–8.4	2.6	70	14
Jacobsen et al[28]	156	122 Recal 34 no previous tx	All sites	No	8.0		68% of recal 47 of no previous tx	
Kenton-Smith et al[29]	123	103 Recal 20 no previous tx	All sites		6.0–9.0	2.1 1.6	92 of recal 75 of no previous tx	
Ross et al[30]	96	Recal	All sites	Yes	9.4	3.4	48	31
Robson et al[33]	194		All sites	Yes	9.0–9.5	2.06	66	

Recal, recalcitrant; tx, therapy.

Other studies on warts demonstrated wide-ranging cure rates using the PDL (Table 11.3). For example, when recalcitrant verrucae on various body sites were treated, clearance rates from 48% to 93% were demonstrated. The average number of treatments ranged from 2.1 to 3.4. In addition, periungual and plantar warts had wide response rates ranging from 33% to 83% and 20% to 84% respectively. Palmar warts demonstrated clearance rates of 65–84%.[25–29] Reports in the podiatry literature demonstrate higher success rates of 70–80% for plantar warts treated with the PDL.[30,31] The wide range in reported success rates may be the result of numerous variables, including the type of wart, selection of recalcitrant patient populations with resistant warts, energy fluence, number of pulses at each site, and different treatment intervals.[32]

A prospective randomized trial was performed by Robson et al[32] which compared PDL therapy with conventional therapy (cryotherapy or cantharidin) for treatment of verrucae. All lesions were pared before treatment. Home therapy for all warts was also performed with daily application of salicylic acid under occlusion. Complete resolution after two treatments was noted in 70% of patients treated with conventional methods, compared with 66% of patients treated with PDL. This difference was not statistically significant. Interestingly, response rates did not vary with regard to the location of the lesion. This study concludes that PDL therapy is as effective as conventional therapy in treating warts.[32] Collectively, the data support classifying PDL therapy as level II evidence based on our Modified Evidence-based Medicine System (Chapter 19) since a randomized controlled study demonstrates findings similar to those found in a number of cohort studies.

Favored methodology

The PDL is a less aggressive approach to the destruction of wart tissue than the CO_2 laser.

This laser operates on the principle of selective photothermolysis and thereby causes less destruction of adjacent tissue. Less anesthesia is necessary than with the CO_2 laser. Some patients tolerate this procedure without anesthesia and almost all others do well with topical anesthetic cream applied under occlusion before the procedure.

Pulsed dye lasers are available with 577, 585, 595 600 nm wavelengths. We use a Scleroplus™ laser (Candela Corporation, Wayland, MA) set at 595 nm with a 5-mm spot-size, 1.5-ms pulse duration at a fluence of 10–20 J/cm^2 with a cryogen spray cooling device. This provides a short burst of cryogen immediately before the laser pulse, which cools the epidermis and allows use of a higher fluence. Warts receive one to several pulses per spot and may receive 5–10 pulses in exceptional cases (usually at lower fluences), until hemorrhagic changes are seen in and around the wart. A dressing is usually not necessary and pain medication is very rarely necessary.

Adverse effects and laser safety

The flashlamp PDL (FPDL) is considered to be the safest vascular laser in use today. It is able to target cutaneous blood vessels selectively with minimal risk of collateral thermal injury and subsequent scarring. Hypertrophic scarring and keloids have been reported but they are extremely rare.[33] One study of 500 patients reported no cases of hypertrophic scarring and the incidence of atrophic scarring was less than 0.1%.[34] A teenager who was taking isotretinoin (Accutane™, Hoffman-La Roche Inc., Nutley, NJ, USA) was reported to have developed keloids after treatment for a hemangioma, and therefore caution has been advised when treating patients who are taking retinoids.[35] Purpura is seen immediately after treatment and lasts

1–2 weeks with the FPDL, but has been reduced recently with the introduction of a laser with a longer pulse duration (V Beam™, *Candela Corporation, Wayland, MA*). Pigmentary changes are also common but transitory and may last from 3 to 6 months.[33]

As lasers emit a very intense beam of light, eye protection is of paramount importance with the PDL. This eyewear is specifically designed for the appropriate wavelength and must be worn by everyone in the room. Several incidences of fires occurring during use of PDL for treatment of port-wine stains have been reported.[36,37] The CO_2 laser could also easily cause a conflagration. However, ignition has not been reported during treatment of verrucae. Dry cloth or paper should not be placed in the treatment field, and combustible materials (gauze, drapes) should be moistened. Alcohol-containing wipes should not be used on the skin because residual alcohol could ignite when exposed to a laser beam. Oxygen should not be present in the treatment field and make-up should be removed from the area because these also pose a hazard.[36]

Human papillomavirus DNA has been identified from laser plumes after CO_2 laser treatment of warts. Although similar studies have not been published with regard to the PDL, it seems prudent to wear protective Micropore laser masks and a smoke evacuator should be used to prevent inhalation of viral particles.[33] Surgical gloves should also be worn by the operator or assistants who come in contact with the lesion to be treated.[17] Patient education of possible risks is aided by the use of a handout (Table 11.4).

Cost–benefit considerations

We could find no studies looking at cost-effectiveness of the FPDL in the treatment of warts. As PDLs can cost over $US80 000 they are generally not utilized as first-line treatment of

Table 11.4 Patient education sheet – pulsed dye laser

General information

Laser is an acronym for light amplification by stimulated emission of radiation. This means lasers generate an intense beam of light energy. When this light is absorbed by your skin, heat is generated that destroys blood vessels in your wart. The doctor may recommend a topical anesthetic that is applied 2 hours before the procedure. With each pulse of the laser you may feel a rubberband-like snap against your skin. You will be required to wear special goggles when the laser is in use.

Day of treatment
- Clean warts with soap and water the morning of your treatment
- Tell your doctor if you have any medicine allergies or seizure disorder
- Wear comfortable clothing that can be easily removed to expose the area to be treated
- You will see bright flashes of light during the treatment
- Let your doctor know if you feel any pain during the treatment

Post-treatment instructions
- Apply antibiotic ointment twice daily to the treatment site if the skin crusts or peels
- Cover with a non-stick dressing if the skin is open
- Call your doctor if you have increasing pain, yellow drainage, expanding redness, a red streak, fever, or any other unusual symptoms

warts. It remains an excellent alternative when other modalities have failed, and in cases of multiple or large warts not amenable to less expensive therapy.

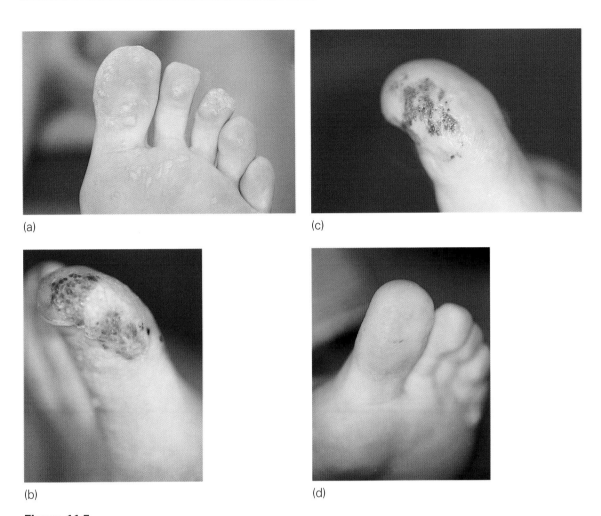

(a)   (c)

(b)   (d)

Figure 11.5
(a) Mosaic warts, 1–4 mm in diameter, over the right big toe, second, third, and fourth toes, and the ball of the foot. (b) Necrotic appearance of the confluent wart on the right big toe 1 week after vascular lesion laser therapy (595 nm). (c) Six weeks after initial therapy, the thick necrotic wart has resolved, leaving superficial crusting, after three treatments with the vascular lesion laser (595 nm). The overall thickness of the wart is markedly decreased. (d) Eight weeks after initial treatment, all the wart has resolved after four treatments with the vascular lesion laser (595 nm).

Case report

A 22-year-old white man presented for evaluation of warts, which had been increasing in number and size over the past 18 months. He had had no previous treatment. Physical examination revealed 35 warts 1–4 mm in diameter on the left foot, with some confluence on the left big toe and left third toe, forming larger mosaic lesions (Figure 11.5a). After discussing costs, risks, and benefits, the patient elected to undergo treatment with the

Table 11.5 Comparison of CO_2 and pulsed dye laser (PDL) in the treatment of warts

	CO_2	PDL
Wavelength (nm)	10 600	585
Target chromophore	Water	Oxyhemoglobin
Power output (W)	10–20	
Energy fluence (J/cm^2)		7–9
Cryogen	No	Yes

vascular lesion laser. Using a power density of 20 J/cm^2, a wavelength of 595 nm, a 5-mm spot size, a pulse duration of 1500 μs with a pulse rate of 1 Hz, and dynamic cooling with liquid nitrogen, the entire exposed surface of wart was treated, hitting each spot with three pulses. Immediately after the treatment the warts showed a slight purpuric appearance. One week later, the warts appeared superficially necrotic over the area of confluent warts on the left big toe, and smaller lesions had sloughed (Figure 11.5b). Treatments were repeated every 2 weeks on three occasions. Two weeks after the third treatment, only superficial crusting was present over the left big toe and the overall thickness of the warts was 90% improved (Figure 11.5c). Two weeks after a fourth and final treatment (8 weeks after initial treatment), all warts had resolved (Figure 11.5d). Six months later the patient returned for follow-up and there were no visible warts. The patient reported that he had only two small recurrent areas of wart on the left foot in the months after his laser surgery, both of which responded to daily home salicylic acid treatments over 10–14 days.

SUMMARY

In summary, both the CO_2 laser and pulsed dye laser have a use in treating warts[38] (Table 11.5). The authors have also had experience using the alexandrite laser (755 nm) for treatment of warts and seborrheic keratoses.[39] The entire surface of warts is treated with 80–100 J/cm^2, spot size 8 mm, without stacking pulses. It remains to be seen whether this approach will be as effective as the CO_2 laser and PDL. The high cost of equipment has hindered the dissemination of all forms of laser technology.

REFERENCES

1. Fairhurst MV, Roenigk RK, Brodland DG. Carbon dioxide laser surgery for skin disease. *Mayo Clin Proc* 1992; **67**: 49–58.
2. Hruza GJ. A novice's guide. *Skin Aging* 2000; **8**: 24–30.
3. Alster TS. *Manual of Cutaneous Laser Techniques*, 2nd edn. Philadelphia: Lippincott Williams & Wilkins, 2000.
4. Alster TS, Lupton JR. Lasers in dermatology. *Am J Clin Dermatol* 2001; **2**: 291–303.
5. Anderson RR, Parrish JA. Selective photothermolysis: precise microsurgery by selective absorption of pulsed radiation. *Science* 1983; **22**: 524–7.
6. Goldman MP, Fitzpatrick RE. *Cutaneous Laser Surgery: The art and science of selective photothermolysis*. St Louis: Mosby Inc., 1999.

7. Mueller TJ, Carlson BA, Lindy MP. The use of the carbon dioxide surgical laser for the treatment of verrucae. *J Am Podiatr Med Assoc* 1980; **70**: 136–41.

8. Logan RA, Zachary CB. Outcome of carbon dioxide laser therapy for persistent cutaneous viral warts. *Br J Dermatol* 1989; **121**: 99–105.

9. Apfelberg DB, Druker D, Masser MR, White DN, Lash H, Spector P. Benefits of the CO_2 laser for verruca resistant to other modalities of treatment. *J Dermatol Surg Oncol* 1989; **15**: 371–5.

10. Sloan K, Haberman H, Lynde CW. Carbon dioxide laser-treatment of resistant verrucae vulgaris: retrospective analysis. *J Cutan Med Surg* 1998; **2**: 142–5.

11. Lim JTE, Goh CL. Carbon dioxide laser treatment of periungual and subungual viral warts. *Aust J Dermatol* 1992; **33**: 87–91.

12. McBurney EI, Rosen DA. Carbon dioxide laser treatment of verrucae vulgares. *J Dermatol Surg Oncol* 1984; **10**: 45–8.

13. Street ML, Roenigk RK. Recalcitrant periungual verrucae: the role of carbon dioxide laser vaporization. *J Am Acad Dermatol* 1990; **23**: 115–20.

14. Silva PD, Micha JP, Silva DG. Management of condyloma acuminatum. *J Am Acad Dermatol* 1985; **13**: 457–63.

15. Bar-Am A, Shilon M, Peyser MR, Ophir J, Brenner S. Treatment of male genital condylomatous lesions by carbon dioxide laser after failure of previous nonlaser methods. *J Am Acad Dermatol* 1991; **24**: 87–9.

16. Dover JS, Arndt KA, Geronemus RG, Alora MBT. Continuous and pulsed carbon dioxide laser surgery. In: *Illustrated Cutaneous and Aesthetic Laser Surgery*, 2nd edn. Stamford, CT: Appleton & Lange, 2000: 35–42.

17. Olbricht SM. Use of the carbon dioxide laser in dermatologic surgery. *J Dermatol Surg Oncol* 1993; **19**: 364–9.

18. Gloster HM, Roenigk RK. Risk of acquiring human papillomavirus from the plume produced by the carbon dioxide laser in the treatment of warts. *J Am Acad Dermatol* 1995; **32**: 436–41.

19. Hughes PSH, Hughes AP. Absence of human papillomavirus DNA in the plume of erbium: YAG laser-treated warts. *J Am Acad Dermatol* 1998; **38**: 426–8.

20. Hallmo P, Naess O. Laryngeal papillomatosis with human papillomavirus DNA contracted by a laser surgeon. *Eur Arch Otorhinolaryngol* 1991; **248**: 425–7.

21. Alam M, Stiller M. Direct medical costs for surgical and medical treatment of condylomata acuminata. *Arch Dermatol* 2001; **137**: 337–41.

22. Strauss MJ, Khanna V, Koenig JD, et al. The cost of treating genital warts. *Int J Dermatol* 1996; **35**: 340–8.

23. Hruza GJ, Geronemus RG, Dover JS, Arndt KA. Lasers in dermatology–1993. *Arch Dermatol* 1993; **129**: 1026–35.

24. Tan OT, Hurwitz RM, Stafford TJ. Pulsed dye laser treatment of recalcitrant verrucae: a preliminary report. *Lasers Surg Med* 1993; **13**: 127–37.

25. Kauvar AN, McDaniel DH, Geronemus RG. Pulsed dye laser treatment of warts. *Arch Fam Med* 1995; **4**: 1035–40.

26. Webster GF, Satur N, Goldman MP, Halmi B, Greenbaum S. Treatment of recalcitrant warts using the pulsed dye laser. *Cutis* 1995; **56**: 230–2.

27. Jacobsen E, McGraw R, McCagh S. Pulsed dye laser efficacy as initial therapy for warts and against recalcitrant verrucae. *Cutis* 1997; **59**: 206–8.

28. Kenton-Smith J, Tan ST. Pulsed dye laser therapy for viral warts. *Br J Plast Surg* 1999; **52**: 554–8.

29. Ross BS, Levine VJ, Nehal K, Tse Y, Ashinoff R. Pulsed dye laser treatment of warts: an update. *Dermatol Surg* 1999; **25**: 377–80.

30. Borovoy MA, Borovoy M, Elson LM, Sage M. Flashlamp pulsed dye laser (585 nm) treatment of resistant verrucae. *J Am Podiatr Med Assoc* 1996; **86**: 547–50.

31. Jain A, Storwick GS. Effectiveness of the

585 nm flashlamp-pulsed tunable dye laser (PTDL) for treatment of plantar verrucae. *Lasers Surg Med* 1997; **21**: 500–5.

32. Robson KJ, Cunningham NM, Kruzan KL, Patel DS, Kreiter CD, O'Donnell MJ. Pulsed-dye laser versus conventional therapy in the treatment of warts: a prospective randomized trial. *J Am Acad Dermatol* 2000; **43**: 275–80.

33. Nanni CA, Alster TS. Complications of cutaneous laser surgery. *Dermatol Surg* 1998; **24**: 209–219.

34. Levine VJ, Geronemus RG. Adverse effects associated with the 577- and 585-nanometer pulsed dye laser in the treatment of cutaneous vascular lesions: a study of 500 patients. *J Am Acad Dermatol* 1995; **32**: 613–17.

35. Bernstein LJ, Geronemus RG. Keloid formation with the 585-nm pulsed dye laser during isotretinoin treatment. *Arch Dermatol* 1997; **133**: 111–12.

36. Waldorf HA, Kauvar ANB, Geronemus RG. Remote fire with the pulsed dye laser: risk and prevention. *J Am Acad Dermatol* 1996; **34**: 503–6.

37. Fretzin S, Beeson WH, Hanke CW. Ignition potential of the 585-nm pulsed dye laser. *Dermatol Surg* 1996; **22**: 699–702.

38. Alster TS, Bettencourt MS. Review of cutaneous lasers and their applications. *South Med J* 1998; **91**: 806–14.

39. Mehrabi D, Brodell RT. Case Report: Use of the alexandrite laser for treatment of seborrheic keratoses. *Dermatol Surg.* 2002; **28**: 437–9.

12 Surgical therapy

Geneviève Fortier-Riberdy and Manish Khanna

Historical aspects • Clinical studies • Case study • Favored treatment methodology • Conclusion • References

A surgical approach to wart treatment seems untenable because the disease is infectious by nature, and affects both abnormal and normal appearing epithelium. Surgical treatments are aimed at destruction or removal of visually infected tissues, with or without a healthy appearing peripheral margin. This chapter discusses cold blade excision of warts, as well as electrosurgery. Some authors noticed a spontaneous resolution of untreated smaller satellite warts after the surgical excision of a predominating wart.[1] One can speculate that a release of antigenic wart material after surgery of a wart stimulates an immune response. This phenomenon is neither constant nor specific to surgical treatment, and it is not well understood. Alternatively, decreasing viral load by debulking a wart may lead to more effective host defences. Finally, debulking may permit more effective treatment by another modality used in combination with surgery.

HISTORICAL ASPECTS

Consequent to the development of effective immunotherapy, surgery for wart treatment will hopefully become obsolete, and be assigned to the history books. It is obviously not a modern or currently popular treatment, as the dates of the references involved in this chapter demonstrate. Most authors recognize that surgery of warts is a potentially morbid and disproportionate method of treatment in relation to the nature of the disease.[2] Until immunotherapy becomes more refined, efficient and specific, however, there are still some situations where a surgical approach to warts may be helpful. Tables 12.1 and 12.2 show the indications and contraindications to such an approach.

Table 12.1 Indications for wart surgery/electrosurgery

Wart resistant to conventional accessible methods
Solitary warts
Filiform warts
Cutaneous horns
Polypoid warts (such as condylomata)

Table 12.2 Relative contraindications for surgery/electrosurgery

Warts in children
Warts on the palms and soles
Multiple warts, especially if they are in a spreading phase
Periungual warts
Warts on the vermillion border of the lip
Warts in an immunosuppressed individual

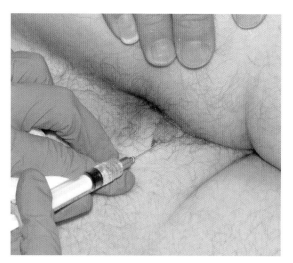

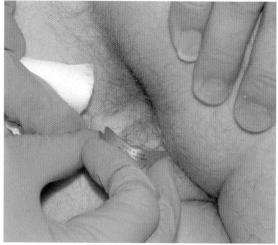

Figure 12.1
A 30-gauge needle is used to infiltrate lignocaine (lidocaine) with adrenaline (epinephrine) around a perianal wart.

Figure 12.2
A sterile razor blade is used to excise (shave) the perianal wart.

CLINICAL STUDIES

Surgery for condylomas

In 1978, Thomson and Grace[3] published a study describing a 'new' operative technique for perianal and anal condyloma treatment. In their article, they suggested that surgeons should abandon extensive ablative electrosurgery for genital condylomata, in order to avoid surgical complications such as anal strictures and deformity. Instead, they recommend using sharp-pointed scissors to remove the lesions, after locally infiltrating the area with an adrenaline (epinephrine) solution (their patients being under general anesthesia). The infiltration permits separation of individual lesions from one another, which helps to preserve healthy skin and accelerates healing. Hemostasis very rarely required electrocoagulation in their series. A total of 75 patients were treated for perianal and anal condylomas as described above and 58%

obtained a cure with a follow-up from 3 to 12 months. A 'minimal recurrence', defined as less than five small condylomas readily controlled with podophyllin application, was observed in 16% of their patients. Finally, 23% necessitated further operative removal of condylomas to obtain a cure and 3% could not be controlled by operative means. The authors conclude that, in three out of four patients, their technique was followed by no significant wart recurrence. With the ever-increasing trend towards ambulatory care, many physicians perform this kind of procedure under local anesthesia with lidocaine (lignocaine) and epinephrine (adrenaline) (Figures 12.1, 12.2 and 12.3).

In 1991, Handley and collegues[4] published a study that presents scissor excision and electrosurgery performed under brief general anaesthesia as a simple, safe and human alternative to unsuccessful outpatient measures in children with persistent or relentlessly progressive anogenital warts.

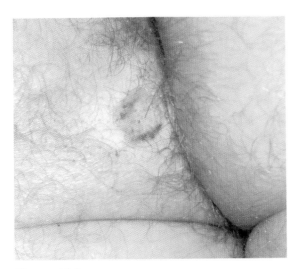

Figure 12.3
Aspect of the wound bed immediately postoperatively.

cially (Walden blunt dissector or Penfield dissector). Alternatively, one could use a nail elevator, an open curette or a closed curette (spoon shaped). The technique permits enucleation of the wart (also termed 'exchocliation' in the podiatric literature[6]), leaving the dermis practically intact, which is favorable for the postoperative healing process. Electrodessication was not used after the wart excision in this series, which probably also contributes to faster healing and less scar formation. Other authors have advocated this type of procedure for plantar warts.[5-8]

The strength of the recommendations supporting the use of surgery for plantar warts is level V according to our Modified Evidence-based Medicine system (see Chapter 19).

Electrosurgery for condylomas

For anogenital condylomas, electrosurgery was compared with CO_2 laser ablation in a study by Ferenczy et al[9] published in 1995. This open clinical trial included 208 observable patients (135 women and 73 men). The authors treated half the lesions in each patient with electrosurgery and the other half with CO_2 laser. All the patients were followed for a mean of 8 months after the last treatment received. Patients with extensive disease and those with intra-anal involvement were treated under general anesthesia. In the remainder of the patients, treatment was done under local anesthesia. Severe discomfort occurred in 12% of patients and 4% developed delayed complications such as hypopigmentation and scarring, irrespective of the treatment modalities used. Complete clearance of condylomata was similar in areas treated with electrosurgery and CO_2 laser. A single treatment cleared 51% of the women and 38% of the men. After four treatments, 75% of the women and 64% of the men were cleared. In this study, clearance was significantly higher for patients whose total condylomatous area

The strength of the recommendations supporting the use of surgery for condylomas can be estimated using evidence-based medicine techniques. We determined that the level of evidence is V according to our Modified Evidence-based Medicine system (see Chapter 19).

Surgery for plantar warts

In 1973 Pringle and Helms[1] published a study including 58 patients treated with 'blunt dissection' for plantar warts. Their cure rate was 85%, after a follow-up period averaging 10 months (minimum of 6 months). As a result of their technique, none of the patients developed painful scar formation. The characteristic of this technique was to avoid using a sharp instrument to perform the wart dissection. Instead, a scalpel handle (modified by the authors to give the tip a curvature) was used. This type of instrument is available commer-

did not exceed 5 cm^2, had not been treated previously for a year or longer, who had condylomata that were in non-anal sites and who were exclusively heterosexual males.

In a study by Stone et al,[10] 71% of patients who received up to six weekly electrosurgical treatments ($n = 88$) obtained complete clearance of their external genital warts at a 3- to 5-month follow-up visit. Simmons et al[11] treated 18 male patients with electrosurgery for genital warts and followed 11 at 3 months, with a cure observed in 10 (90% of observable patients).

With regard to the preoperative local anesthesia, some authors studied the use of EMLA (eutectic mixture of local anesthetics) cream alone and showed good results. Lunghall and Lillieborg[12] found that EMLA cream applied by medical staff in a thick layer, under occlusion, 5–10 minutes before electrosurgery of vulvar condylomata provided satisfactory anaesthesia in 92% of the women treated ($n = 42$). Interestingly, the analgesic efficacy decreased gradually with application times of 15 minutes and longer. A previous study had shown that EMLA cream was effective only in 40% of women treated for genital condylomata, but these poor results seem to be related to the excessive length of application times (30–105 minutes).[13]

The strength of the recommendations supporting the use of electrosurgery and curettage for warts is level III according to our Modified Evidence-based Medicine system (see Chapter 19).

Electrosurgery and curettage of warts

In a retrospective study published in 1969, Baar and Coles[14] showed that the combination of electrosurgery and curettage in 46 patients with hand warts yielded a success rate of 80%. In the same study, electrosurgery alone gave a 62% cure rate in 21 patients, and curettage alone gave a cure rate of 58% in 71 patients.

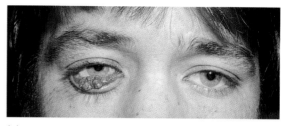

(a)

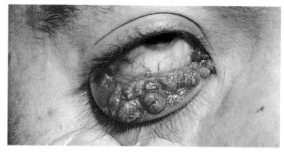

(b)

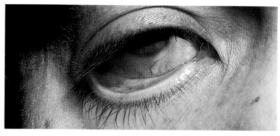

(c)

Figure 12.4

(a) A large verrucous growth is present on the palpebral conjunctiva of the right lower eyelid prior to treatment. (b) A closer view of the lesion before treatment demonstrates confluent pin-point to 3 mm diameter papules with fine surface projections and scale crusting in this broad plaque-like lesion. (c) Healed conjunctiva with minimal scarring and no recurrent wart is noted 5 months after excision followed ny liquid-nitrogen cryotherapy of the lesion pictured above. *Reprinted with permission of Ophthalmic Surgery from Miller DM, Brodell RT, Levine MR, The Conjunctival Wart: Report of a Case and Review of Treatment Options, Ophthal Surg, 1994;25:545–548.

Unfortunately, the details of treatment methods were not described, the follow-up period was not mentioned and the incidence of postoperative scarring was not addressed. Another retrospective study published in 1978 assessed the cure rate after electrosurgery and curettage of warts located mainly on the hands, and found a 95% cure rate with a mean follow-up period of 12.7 years. Similar limitations were present in this study.[15]

CASE STUDY

A 33-year-old man had a history of a wart removed from his right lower eyelid. He had no prior history of warts or other human papillomavirus (HPV) infections. Eight months later, the patient noted a wart adjacent to the excision site. The wart interfered with eyelid closure, leading to recurrent conjunctivitis. The patient presented to the dermatology clinic. On physical examination, a 2.5 × 1 cm pink, friable, fixed, verrucous growth was found emanating from the palpebral conjunctiva of the right lower eyelid and extending into the lower fornix. After careful ophthalmological evaluation, the lesion was excised to tarsus and Tenon's capsule. The base and surrounding conjunctiva were then treated with cryotherapy to –30°C for 25 seconds. The patient has remained wart-free for 5 months (Figure 12.4). (See Miller et al[16] for a complete description of this case.

FAVORED TREATMENT METHODOLOGY

Electrosurgery

1. Injection of local anesthetics with epinephrine (adrenaline) when the location is not contraindicated
2. Destruction of the visible wart tissue with electrodessication to produce a white color, with some charring on top
3. Curettage to scoop out the burned tissue with a ring curette
4. Dessication can be repeated, followed by curettage, until a healthy appearing tissue is reached at the base of the wound
5. If a palm or a sole is treated, scissors are used to trim the excess hyperkeratotic tissue present at the periphery of the lesion

Surgery for condylomas

1. For vulvar and perianal condylomas, the lithotomy position is ideal but, if the physician prefers, the jack-knife position can be used
2. Injection of local anesthetics with epinephrine (adrenaline), when the location is not contraindicated. Following the injection the condylomas tend to separate
3. With a pair of fine-toothed forceps and fine-pointed scissors, the condylomas are individually excised, preserving as much normal skin as possible in between. The excision can also be made with a sterile razor blade held in a curved shape between the first and second or third finger (shave excision)
4. There is usually little bleeding, but electrocautery may occasionally be needed
5. It is not always possible to remove all lesions in one intervention, because of the extent of the disease and the risk of postoperative strictures. In this event, a 1-month interval is suggested before further treatment

Enucleation of plantar warts

1. Superficial callus and warty tissue is pared until the sharp demarcation between the wart and normal surrounding skin is clear

Table 12.3 Patient education sheet: postoperative care after surgery of a wart

1. The wound should be washed with soap and water twice daily, followed by hydrogen peroxide cleansing
2. An antibiotic ointment or petrolatum jelly can be applied twice daily under a Telfa adhesive bandage
3. The wound will usually heal in 2–3 weeks and possibly leave a flat permanent white scar

2. Local anesthesia is first administered by a Dermo-Jet (Robbins Instruments Inc., Chatham, NJ), followed by infiltration with a 25-gauge needle under the wart and then superficially on each side of the wart
3. Using a blunt dissector instrument (see text), the wart is encircled using firm pressure and a peeling motion to separate the wart from the peripheral tissue
4. The callused margins of the wound are trimmed with curved scissors
5. The wound is covered with a pressure dressing which is replaced with a conventional bandage 2 days after the procedure

A patient information sheet can be helpful (Table 12.3).

CONCLUSION

In certain clinical settings, a surgical approach to warts will be desirable and suitable. These indications are summarized in Table 12.1 and include warts that are resistant to conventional accessible methods, solitary warts, filiform warts, cutaneous horns, and polypoid warts. As a result of the difficulty sometimes encountered in differentiating a wart from a hypertrophic actinic keratosis or a squamous cell carcinoma, a solitary wart on photoexposed skin or in an immunosuppressed patient should be shaved for biopsy.

REFERENCES

1. Pringle WM, Helms DC. Treatment of plantar warts by blunt dissection. *Arch Dermatol* 1973; **108**: 79–82.
2. Rook A., Wilkinson DS, Ebling FJG, eds. *Textbook of Dermatology*, 6th edn. Oxford: Blackwell Science, 1998.
3. Thomson JPS, Grace RH. The treatment of perianal and anal condylomata acuminate: a new operative technique. *J R Soc Med* 1978; **71**: 180–5.
4. Handley JM, Maw RD, Horner T et al. Scissor excision plus electrocauthery of anogenital warts in prepubertal children. *Pediatr Dermatol* 1991; **8**: 243–5
5. Prazak G, Thomas DE. Curettage treatment of plantar warts. *Arch Dermatol* 1955; **71**: 122–3.
6. McCarthy DJ. Therapeutic considerations in the treatment of pedal verrucae. *Clin Podiatr Med Surg* 1986; **3**: 433–48.
7. Davidson MR, Schuler BS. Skin curette and the treatment of plantar verrucae. *J Am Podiatr Assoc* 1976; **66**: 331–6.
8. McGregor RR, Wehr GV. Blunt dissection of plantar verrucae using a new instrument. *J Am Podiatr Assoc* 1974; **64**: 92–6.
9. Ferenczy A, Behelak Y, Haber G, Wright TC et al. Treating vaginal and external anogenital condylomas with electrosurgery vs CO_2 laser ablation. *J Gynecol Surg* 1995; **11**: 41–50.
10. Stone KM, Becker TM, Hadgu A, Krauss SJ. Treatment of external genital warts: a randomized clinical trail comparing podophyllin, cryotherapy, and electrodesiccation. *Genitourin Med* 1990; **66**: 16–19.
11. Simmons PD, Langlet F, Thin RNT. Cryotherapy versus electrocautery in the treatment of genital warts. *Br J Vener Dis* 1981; **57**: 273–4.

12. Ljunghall K, Lillieborg S. Local anesthesia with lidocaine/prilocaine cream (EMLA[R]) for cautery of condylomata acuminate on the vulval mucosa. *Arch Derm Venereol* 1989; **69**: 362–5.

13. Hallen A, Ljunghall, Wallin J. Topical anaesthesia with local anaesthetic (lidocaine and prilocaine, EMLA) cream for cautery of genital warts. *Genitourin Med* 1987; **63**: 316–19.

14. Barr A, Coles RB. Warts on the hands. *Trans St John's Hosp Dermatol Soc* 1969; **55**: 69–73.

15. Gibbs RC, Scheiner AM. Long-term follow-up evaluation of patients with electrosurgically treated warts. *Cutis* 1978; **21**: 383–4.

16. Miller DM, Brodell RT, levine MR. The conjunctival wart: report of a case and review of treatment options. *Ophthalmol Surg* 1994; **25**: 545–8..

13 Interferons in the treatment of viral warts

Kyle L Wagamon IV and Robert T Brodell

Historical aspects • Classification • Basic science • Clinical studies • Favored treatment methodology • Adverse effects • Cost–benefit considerations • Case reports • References

Interferons are a family of naturally occurring proteins that act to make cells resistant to viral infection. Their discovery in the 1950s stimulated great interest in the medical and scientific communities because, for the first time, physicians had a method of treating patients with viral infections. Although interferons have shown promising results in treating several different types of viral infections, they are approved by the Food and Drug Administration (FDA) only for the treatment of chronic hepatitis B, chronic hepatitis C, hairy cell leukemia, Kaposi's sarcoma and genital warts. In this chapter, the viability of interferon therapy in the treatment of warts is reviewed.

HISTORICAL ASPECTS

For centuries, scientists and the medical community have recognized two important facts about viral infections: first, a single organism is only rarely infected by two different viruses at one time and, second, once an animal has been infected by a virus it is more difficult to infect that animal with a different virus. These two phenomena were explained in 1957 when two British scientists called Isaacs and Lindenmann began experimenting with virally infected cell cultures. Through their experiments, they discovered that virally infected cells secrete a soluble substance which acts to make normal cells resistant to viral infection. They appropriately named the unknown substance interferon, based on the fact that it acted to interfere with viral replication. Over the next few decades, several different proteins were isolated that had antiviral activity. All of these were included under the interferon name, creating the modern-day family of proteins we know as interferons.

CLASSIFICATION

Today, the interferon family includes many proteins that have been broken down into two broad classes: type I interferons and type II interferons. The type I interferon class includes two groups: α and β. The type II interferon class includes only one group – γ. The α group is secreted by macrophages and is made up of 14 different subtypes, and the γ class is secreted by T lymphocytes and is made up of only a single subtype. Numerous other methods of classification have been applied to the interferons, such as acid stability and cell of origin. However, the underlying feature of these proteins is that they all act to make cells resistant to viral infection.

immune response to attack the virus more efficiently.

BASIC SCIENCE

After isolating the proteins within the interferon family, scientists began to uncover how they work. This subject is still a matter for ongoing research. It is believed that, when a virus binds to its specific receptor on the target cell membrane, a signal is sent to the target cell nucleus, which acts to stimulate the transcription of genes that code for interferon proteins. The interferon proteins are then packaged into tiny vesicles and secreted into the extracellular environment. Within the extracellular environment, the interferons diffuse to the surface of a nearby cell and bind to a specific receptor on its cell membrane. This binding causes a signal to be sent to the cell nucleus, which acts to stimulate the transcription of genes that code for specific proteins. These specific proteins have one of three functions: antiviral activity, antiproliferative activity and immunomodulatory activity. The antiviral proteins are believed to act by seeking out and destroying molecules within the cell that have features specific to viruses such as double-stranded RNA or single-stranded DNA. The antiproliferative proteins act to remove the cell from the growth cycle via an unknown mechanism thereby preventing it from dividing and further replicating the virus. The immunomodulatory proteins act either to stimulate or to inhibit immune function by affecting T lymphocytes, B lymphocytes and natural killer (NK) cells. By stimulating the immune system, virally infected cells are more likely to be destroyed. Hence, all of the proteins that cells synthesize in response to exposure to interferons act to do one of the following: make the cell more resistant to viral infection, reduce proliferation of the cell in case it is already infected or regulate the

CLINICAL STUDIES

In view of the antiviral and antiproliferative activity of interferons, it was believed that they would be an ideal treatment for human papilloma virus infections in humans. The first clinical trials performed in the early 1980s showed promising results. One of the earliest studies was presented at the International Conference on Clinical Potential of Interferons in Viral Diseases and Malignant Tumors held in December of 1980 and was titled 'Interferon treatment of viral warts and some skin diseases'.[1] Both common and genital warts were treated with intralesional injections of interferon with positive results. This and several other studies encouraged a wave of research during the mid to late 1980s, focusing on interferons in the treatment of warts.[2–4] Several randomized controlled trials emerged which assessed the success of treating common and genital warts with both intralesional and systemic interferon therapy. A pivotal randomized controlled trial was performed by Friedman-Kien et al[5] In this study 158 people were randomly assigned to an experimental group and a control group. Patients assigned to the experimental group were given twice-weekly intralesional injections of interferon-αn3 (Alferon N Injection) whereas patients assigned to the control group were given twice-weekly intralesional injections of placebo for up to 8 weeks. Of the patients receiving the interferon-αn3 injections, 62% had a complete remission of their warts during the 8-week treatment period compared with only 21% of the patients receiving placebo. The recurrence rate in the patients receiving interferon was found to be 24%. In addition, results showed that 100% of the patients receiving the interferon-αn3 injections demonstrated improvement of their warts during the 8-week treatment period, compared with only 20% of the patients receiving placebo.

Like the Friedman-Kien study, other double-masked placebo-controlled studies such as those by Eron et al,[2] Vance et al[3] and Welander et al[4] showed that interferon therapy is a viable method for treating both common and genital warts, and is associated with relatively low recurrence rates. However, the results of the studies on systemic interferon therapy were less promising. Most showed only little or no effect of the systemic interferon when compared with placebo.[7–10] The end-result was the FDA approval during the late 1980s of the treatment for persistent or recurrent genital warts that fail to respond to first-line caustic or ablative therapies with intralesional interferon therapy.

Today, there are two different forms of commercial interferon on the market approved for the treatment of persistent/recurrent genital warts. The first is a natural form of a mixture of α interferons purified from human white blood cells called interferon-αn3. The second is a single interferon-α synthesized via recombinant DNA technology, called interferon-α2b (Intron A). Both forms have proved to be effective at treating persistent genital warts, showing a complete clearance of the warts in 47–62% of patients depending on the duration and type of interferon-α used. No comparison studies between the two different forms of commercially available interferon have yet been performed. Studies also revealed that interferon therapy is associated with a low rate of wart recurrence (20–25%) when compared with other more conventional wart treatments. Clearing/shrinkage of the warts can usually be seen after only 3–4 weeks of treatment, depending on the size and number of the given lesions. However, those patients treated should receive therapy for 8 weeks before a different treatment modality is attempted. Treatment of warts with a combination of inter-ferons and laser, interferons and retinoids, etc. is promising but requires further study before being implemented.[8–12]

The strength of the recommendations supporting the use of interferons in the treatment of warts can be estimated using evidence-based medicine techniques. According to our Modified Evidence-based Medicine System (see Chapter 19), the use of interferon for ano-genital warts is supported by evidence rated level I. This is justified because the treatment is supported by several large randomized clinical trials.[13]

FAVORED TREATMENT METHODOLOGY

The most significant procedural difference between the two commercially available interferons is that the recombinant interferon product (interferon-α2b) is recommended three times each week, whereas the natural interferon product (interferon-αn3) is recommended two times each week. Recommended protocols are as follows: the intralesional dosage for the recombinant interferon (interferon-α2b) is 0.1 ml (1×10^6 IU) per wart with a maximum dose of 0.5 ml (5×10^6 IU) per treatment session, whereas the intralesional dosage for the natural interferon product (interferon-αn3) is 0.05 ml (250×10^3 IU) per wart with a maximum dose of (2.5×10^6 IU) per treatment session (Table 13.1).

Intralesional interferon should be administered as follows: EMLA (eutectic mixture of local anesthetics) is applied under occlusive dressing to the target area 1 hour before the patient is scheduled to undergo treatment. A 30-gauge needle is then inserted parallel to the surface of the skin immediately adjacent to the wart and directed towards the wart's center. The injected interferon should produce a raised weal similar to a correctly administered purified protein derivative (PPD) test. This technique

Table 13.1 Interferon treatment methodology

Interferon type	No. of treatments/week	Dose/wart (ml)	Maximum dose/ session (ml)
Interferon-α2b (Intron)	3	0.1	0.5
Interferon-αn3 (Alferon)	2	0.05	0.5

ensures that the medication is delivered to the vicinity of the virally infected cells. Most patients have tolerated the injections well and even prefer the injections to the pain associated with other caustic or ablative treatment methods. One unique method of administering interferons that requires further study is via needleless injector, a medical tool that uses high pressure to inject substances directly through the skin. One study[14] found the needleless injector to be a successful means of administering interferon therapy as opposed to using regular injections. After a full treatment course, it is wise to wait at least 8 weeks to see whether improvement continues into the post-treatment period before attempting another mode of therapy.

ADVERSE EFFECTS

Adverse affects to interferons are mild and most often include local reaction at the injection site and flu-like symptoms. Local reactions include erythema, edema, bleeding and rare cases of ulceration. Flu-like symptoms include fever, chills, headache, fatigue, malaise and myalgias. Most of the flu-like symptoms can be relieved with acetaminophen (paracetamol) after treatment and last only a short period of time after the injection. In addition, as patients continue with treatment, the flu-like symptoms tend to decrease in intensity, often tapering off completely. Some studies have reported elevations in serum lipids in people being treated

Table 13.2 Adverse effects of interferons

Local reaction:
   Erythema
   Edema
   Bleeding
   Rare ulceration
Flu-like symptoms:
   Fever
   Chills
   Headache
   Fatigue
   Malaise
   Myalgias

with interferons. However, these studies all dealt with patients receiving systemic interferon injections and not intralesional ones as in the case of wart treatment (Table 13.2). A patient education sheet can be helpful (Table 13.3).

COST–BENEFIT CONSIDERATIONS

A major consideration when contemplating interferon as a treatment for warts is cost. When discussing cost, one must include both direct and indirect costs. Recent publications list the direct cost of interferon-α at about $US6 per injection. This means that interferon therapy can cost from $US180 to $US1200 or

Table 13.3 Patient education sheet

What are interferons?
Interferons are a family of naturally occurring proteins that act to make cells resistant to viral infections. By making your cells resistant to infection, they act to prevent the wart virus from multiplying within your body. However, remember that warts are not easy to treat. It will take several treatment sessions to get rid of warts and there is no guarantee that this method of treatment will work for you.

1. **Before treatment:**
   - Interferon treatments are administered via series of injections using a very small, 30-gauge needle. Although this sounds painful, you may prefer this method of treatment when compared to other treatments, such as freezing, surgery or acids. EMLA is a prescription product that should be applied one hour before the injections to reduce the pain of the needle sticks.
   - Interferons are associated with mild non-life-threatening side effects, such as local reactions around the injection site and flu-like symptoms. The flu-like symptoms can often be treated with a single dose of acetaminophen (paracetamol) 325 mg, 1 hour after the injections.
2. **During treatment:**
   - You will feel a needle being inserted into the warts.
   - Tell your doctor about any changes associated with the injection site during the period immediately after injection.
3. **After treatment:**
   - Call the physician if you have any problems with fever, expanding reaction around the injection site, or resistant pain.
   - Remember, do not be upset if the warts do not go away with one or a few treatments.
   - Warts can come back even after they appear to have cleared completely. Please call your physician with any signs of recurrence.

more depending on the duration of the treatment and the number of lesions being treated. Other direct costs include physician visits, which would be up to $US1000 if treatment lasts 8 weeks. However, the high direct costs associated with interferon therapy are offset by the relatively low indirect costs, e.g. interferons do not require any post-treatment wound care, pain medication, sleep medication or absenteeism from work. Of particular importance is the fact that interferon-α of all types is associated with a lower rate of wart recurrence than other more traditional wart treatments. Therefore, choosing interferon therapy may be more cost-effective than attempting to treat a patient with multiple alternative caustic or ablative techniques. In conclusion, interferons are a viable therapy for patients with resistant viral warts that have not responded to other more conventional treatments.

CASE REPORTS

Case 1

A 43-year-old man presented with an 8-month history of perianal warts. He had previously been treated on multiple occasions with liquid

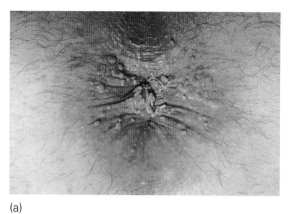

(a)

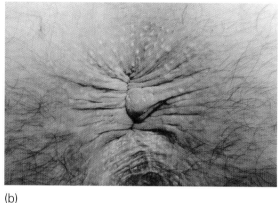

(b)

Figure 13.1

(a) Before intralesional interferon treatment. Dozens of 0.2–1 mm diameter perianal warts have resisted therapy with multiple treatments with liquid nitrogen cryotherapy, 2 months of podophyllin home treatment, and CO_2 laser ablation on two occasions. (b) After intralesional interferon-α treatment. Complete clearing of all warts following biweekly intralesional treatment with 0.05 ml to each wart for a total of 0.5 ml per treatment after 5 weeks.

nitrogen, podophyllum and cold steel surgery, with incomplete clearing or prompt recurrence after each therapeutic maneuver. Physical examination revealed dozens of 0.5- to 1.5-mm condylomata accuminata in the perianal region (Figure 13.1a). Education about the nature of the disease was provided to the patient and the risks and benefits of interferon therapy were discussed. Interferon therapy was initiated using the natural interferon, interferon-αn3, as per standard protocol receiving two doses each week. Within 5 weeks he showed excellent improvement, with only five or six 0.1-mm warts remaining. Within 6 weeks only three pinpoint warts remained and by 7 weeks the warts had cleared completely (Figure 13.1b). The patient was then referred to a gastroenterologist for sigmoidoscopy and no internal warts were found. The patient has not had any recurrence after 4 years.

Case 2

A 39-year-old woman presented with a 1-year history of perianal and vulvar warts. She had received biweekly podophyllum treatment for 10 weeks in the past with no improvement. Physical examination showed confluent cauliflower-like masses of warts in the perianal area and one smaller wart on the labia majora (Figure 13.2a). After discussing available treatment modalities, including CO_2 laser, intralesional interferon, continued podophyllum, acid and liquid nitrogen, intralesional interferon was chosen. Two doses of natural interferon, interferon-αn3, were administered each week for the next 8 weeks. Definite improvement was first noticed after 3 weeks of treatment (Figure 13.2b). The warts continued to improve with further treatment and were noted to have cleared completely by the end of the treatment

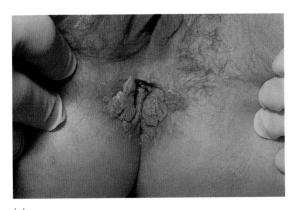

(a)

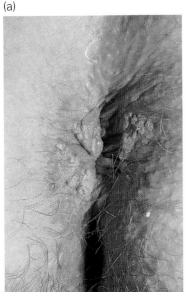

(b)

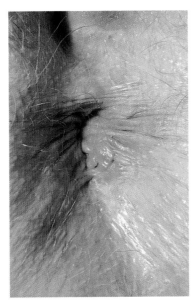

(c)

Figure 13.2
(a) Before intralesional interferon-α treatment: cauliflower-like perianal warts are present which have never been treated. (b) Four weeks after intralesional interferon-α treatment; 0.5–2 mm warts remain, but overall show 75% improvement with biweekly intralesional interferon-α treatments using 0.05 ml injected into 10 foci with each intralesional treatment. Injection sites were rotated so that all areas were treated over time. (c) Seven weeks after intralesional interferon-α treatment, all warts are entirely cleared. Treatment was discontinued and no warts recurred over the follow-up period of 2 years.

period (Figure 13.2c). The patient was seen on three additional occasions over the next 2 years with no recurrence of warts. Annual Papanicolaou smears have been negative.

Case 3

A 12-year-old girl presented for evaluation of two warts on her right (dominant) hand. These had been present for 6 weeks and over the past 2 weeks had rapidly increased in size. Her medical history was otherwise unremarkable and no other treatment methods had been used at home. Physical examination revealed an 8 × 6 mm verruca on the palmar aspect of the right index finger at the distal interphalangeal joint (Figure 13.3a) and a 2 × 2 mm verruca located on the palmar aspect of the right third finger (not shown). The patient was a pitcher for a local championship softball team

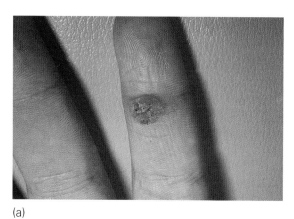
(a)

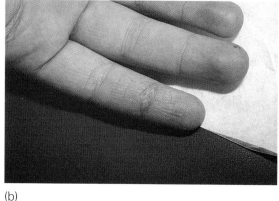
(b)

Figure 13.3

(a) Before intralesional treatment with interferon-α using a Dermo-Jet. A 1 cm diameter verruca is present on the right index finger of a 12-year-old softball pitcher. (b) After intralesional treatment with interferon-α using a Dermo-Jet. The lesion completely resolved after 6 biweekly treatments.

and refused any kind of treatment that might interfere with her pitching over the next 8-week period. Education about the nature of the disease was provided to the patient, and the risks and benefits of interferon therapy were discussed. Treatment was initiated using biweekly intralesional injections of the natural interferon, interferon-αn3. However, because of the patient's fear of needles the interferon was administered using a needleless injector (Dermo-Jet needleless high-pressure injector, Robbins Instruments Inc., Chatham, NJ). After a week of treatment there was visible regression of both verrucae with complete resolution occurring after 3 weeks of treatment (Figure 13.3b).

approximately 1 × 2 cm just lateral to the ball of the left foot (Figure 13.4c). He was treated with a vascular lesion laser for eight treatments – Aldara biweekly for 8 weeks, salicylic acid daily for 6 months, and cantharidin plus salicylic acid plus podophyllin for six treatments for a period of 1 year with only transient improvement. The risks and benefits of interferon therapy were then discussed and treatment was initiated using biweekly intralesional injections of the natural interferon, interferon-αn3. After 7 weeks of treatment, the warts on his hands were completely gone (Figure 13.4b) and the wart on the ball of his left foot was almost completely resolved as well (Figure 13.4d). Two months later all warts had cleared.

Case 4

A 16-year-old boy presented for evaluation of cutaneous warts on the ball of his left foot and right thumb. Physical examination showed four 4-mm diameter warts on the right thumb (Figure 13.4a) and one large mosaic wart measuring

Case 5

A 40-year-old woman presented with a large plantar wart on her left foot. One year ago the wart was treated with CO_2 laser vaporization. Over the past 4 months the wart had rapidly increased in size and was now causing her

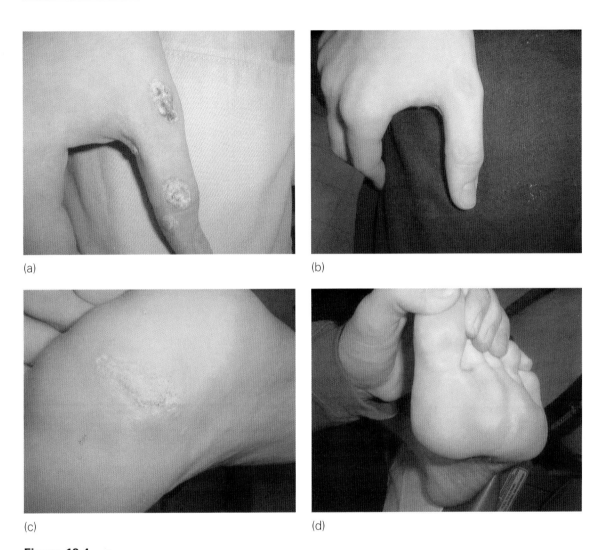

Figure 13.4
(a) Before treatment with interferon-α. Four verrucae are present on the right thumb. All of these lesions have been previously treated with cantharidin, home salicylic acid, Aldara and a vascular lesion laser. (b) Right hand after 7 weeks of intralesional injections with interferon-α. Photograph shows complete clearing of warts with some postinflammatory hyperpigmentation. (c) Before treatment with interferon-α. One large mosaic wart is located lateral to the ball of the foot. (b) Left foot after 7 weeks of intralesional injections with interferon-α. Photograph shows approximately 80% improvement from initial presentation.

significant discomfort whenever she put pressure on it. During the past 3 months, the wart had been treated with liquid nitrogen and cantharidin plus salicylic acid plus podophyllin on a weekly basis, and topical salicylic acid plasters daily. Physical examination showed a 1.8 × 1.2 cm mosaic plantar wart on the left foot at the base of the first metatarsal

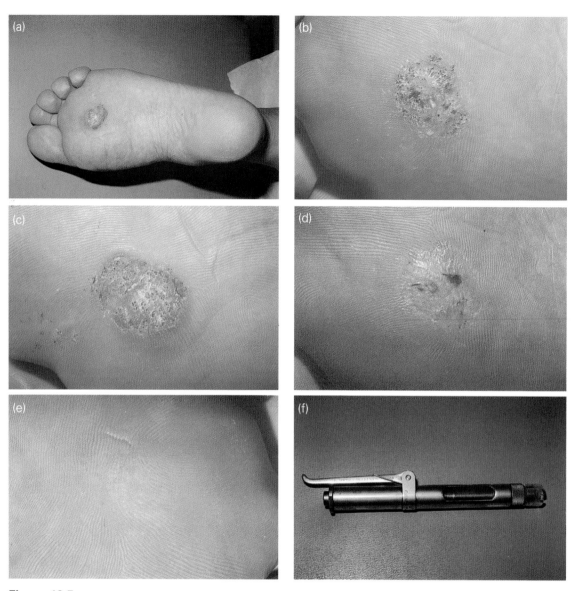

Figure 13.5

(a) Before intralesional treatment with interferon-α using a Dermo-Jet. A 3-cm diameter verruca is present on the sole of the foot. This lesion has resisted therapy with liquid nitrogen cryotherapy, cantharidin, home salicylic acid and CO_2 laser ablation on two occasions. (b) Close-up view of the lesion pictured in (a). (c) Four weeks after intralesional treatment. The lesion is flatter, but continues to show verrucous surface features and thrombosed capillaries. (d) Seven weeks after intralesional treatment, several 0.5 mm foci show slight verrucous surface change and interruption of dermatoglyphs. (e) Six months later with no further treatment. Complete clearing with dermatoglyphs passing through the area previously involved with wart. (f) The Dermo-Jet instrument used in the above treatments. (Reproduced with permission from Naples et al[15])

phalangeal joint (Figure 13.5a, b) no other verrucae were noted. The risks and benefits of interferon therapy were discussed and treatment was initiated using biweekly intralesional injections of the natural interferon, interferon-αn3. The injections were administered using a needleless injector because of the size of the lesions and the patient's anxiety associated with the failed destructive techniques used in the past. Signs of regression of the wart were noted after the first 4 weeks of treatment (Figure 13.5c). Continued resolution of the wart was also noted at 7 weeks (Figure 13.5d) at which point intralesional interferon was discontinued. The wart continued to improve even without therapy as seen at a 6-month follow-up visit where complete resolution of the wart was noted (Figure 13.5e).

REFERENCES

1. Interferon treatment of viral warts and some skin diseases. The clinical potential of interferons: treatment of viral diseases and malignant tumors. *Proceedings of the International Conference on Clinical Potentials of Interferons in Viral Diseases and Malignant Tumors*. Japan Medical Research Foundation Publication No 15. Tokyo, Japan. Dec 2–4, 1980; 149–65.
2. Eron LJ, Judson F, Tucker S et al. Interferon therapy for condylomata acuminata. *N Engl J Med* 1986; **315**: 1059–64.
3. Corwin Vance J, Bart BJ, Hansen RC et al. Intralesional recombinant alpha-2 interferon for the treatment of patients with condyloma acuminatum or verruca planteris. *Arch Dermatol* 1986; **22**: 272–7.
4. Niimura M. Intralesional human fibroblast interferon in common warts. *J Dermatol* 1983; **10**: 217–20.
5. Friedman-Kien AE, Eron LJ, Conant M et al. Natural interferon alfa for treatment of condylomata acuminata. *JAMA* 1988; **259**: 533–8.
6. Welander CE, Homesley HD, Smiles KA, Peets EA. Intralesional interferon alfa-2b for the treatment of genital warts. *Am J Obstet Gynecol* 1990; **162**: 348–54.
7. Condylomata International Collaborative Study Group. Recurrent condylomata acuminata treated with recombinant interferon alfa-2a. *JAMA* 1991; **265**: 2684–7.
8. Condylomata International Collaborative Study Group. Randomized placebo-controlled double-blind combined therapy with laser surgery and systemic interferon alfa-2a in the treatment of anogenital condylomata acuminatum. *J Infect Dis* 1993; **167**: 824–9.
9. Armstrong DKB, Maw RD, Dinsmore WW et al. Combined therapy trial with interferon alpha-2a and ablative therapy in the treatment of anogenital warts. *Genitourin Med* 1996; **72**: 103–7.
10. Armstrong DKB, Maw RD, Dinsmore WW et al. A randomized, double-blind, parallel group study to compare subcutaneous interferon alpha-2a plus podophyllin with placebo plus podophyllin in the treatment of primary condylomata acuminata. *Genitourin Med* 1994; **70**: 389–3.
11. Petersen CS, Bjerring P, Larson J et al. Systemic interferon alpha-2b increases the cure rate in laser treated patients with multiple persistent genital warts: A placebo controlled study. *Genitourin Med* 1991; **67**: 99–102.
12. Cardamakis E, Michopoulos J, Kotoulas IG et al. Comparative study of systemic interferon alfa-2a plus isotretinoin versus isotretinoi in the treatment of recurrent condyloma acuminatum in men. *Urology* 1995; **45**: 857–60.
13. Sterling JC, Handfield-Jones S, Hudson PM. Guidelines for the management of cutaneous warts. *Br J Dermatol* 2001; **144**: 4–11.
14. Naples SP, Brodell RT. Verruca vulgaris. *Arch Dermatol* 1993; **129**: 698–700.

14 Cantharidin

Pradip Bhattacharjee and Robert T Brodell

Historical aspects • Basic science • Clinical studies • Favored treatment methodology • Adverse effects • Cost–benefit considerations • Case reports • References

Cantharidins are purified active ingredients of dried, powdered, blister beetles known as cantharides. It is a lipid-soluble irritant that has the special ability to disorganize epidermal cells and cause subsequent destruction of warts. The history of cantharides use dates back to Greco-Roman times, when it was used to treat a variety of illnesses. More recently, it has been used as an aphrodisiac, abortifacient, and a diuretic agent in veterinary medicine.[1] Interest in the use of this chemical's vesicobullous properties to treat warts began in the early 1900s. In this chapter, the viability of cantharidin therapy in the treatment of warts is reviewed.

HISTORICAL ASPECTS

Many pharmacologic agents have been used throughout the centuries for the treatment of warts. As mentioned above, cantharide use dates back to Greco-Roman times, when it was used to treat a variety of illnesses including dropsy, pleurisy, pericarditis, and amenorrhea.[2] The earliest descriptions of its use as a medicinal agent dates back to 58 BC to AD 29, when the drug was addressed by prominent historical icons in medicine, including Hippocrates, Celsus and Pliny. The drug was advocated by a Greek army physician, Dioscorides, in the first century AD. It was also believed that the Roman Empress Livia was said to have slipped this drug into the food of other members of the imperial family to have them commit sexual indiscretions that could be used against them. It had widespread use during the eighteenth century when it was used to help Louis XV and Ferdinand the Catholic promote stronger sexual desire. During these times, the drug was extracted by the crude methods of directly crushing the dried bodies of blister beetles and mixing them in a solvent.

During the medieval ages, the use of cantharidin was almost non-existent. It was not until 1810 that a French pharmacist, Robiquet,[3] first isolated cantharidins in a crystalline form by dehydration. Subsequently, this compound has been subject to many experiments elucidating its physiologic properties on many organ systems. During the late 1800s, it was well established that this compound was a severe irritant to epithelial linings, including gastrointestinal tract, urinary tract, and skin among other organs.[1] In 1896, Unna[4] showed that cantharidin's primary cutaneous effect was the separation (acantholysis) and death of epidermal cells. Since then, many articles have been published attempting to detail the pathogenic mechanism of the acantholysis of cantharidins.

One of the most publicized effects of cantharidin or 'Spanish fly' in the popular media was that of an aphrodisiac. It was thought that toxic doses of orally administered cantharidin could cause priapism in men and pelvic congestion and uterine bleeding in women.[2] These effects were later found to be caused by the irritant effects of cantharides on the genitourinary tract, which may have been misinterpreted as an increased sensuality. Vichower and Cohen,[5] in 1938, showed that, when cantharidin was dissolved in water and the freshwater crustacean *Daphnia* was put into the solution, the males ejaculated immediately and the females were not affected. Many subsequent reports followed that described serious overdoses of this drug when used orally for its aphrodisiac properties.

Epstein and Kligman[6] authored the first published experiments of using cantharidin topically for the purpose of treating warts in 1958. They had decided to use the acantholytic properties of this compound discovered by Unna and research its use as a chemotherapeutic agent in the treatment of warts. They showed that cantharidin 0.7%, in equal parts of acetone and collodion, when occluded with a Band-Aid, was very effective therapy for common, plantar, and periungual warts. Over the next several decades, many investigators confirmed the usefulness of cantharidin in the treatment of warts. These experiments had brought this chemodestructive modality to the forefront of treatment for human papillomavirus (HPV) infections.

BASIC SCIENCE

Cantharidin is hexahydro-2α, 7α-dimethyl-4-β,7β-epoxyisobenzofura-1,3-dione, the anhydride of cantharidic acid ($C_{10}H_{12}O_4$ or hexahydro-3,7-dimethyl - 4,7-epo-oxyisobenzofuran - 1,3-dione) which is derived from beetles.[1,2] The structure is a bicyclic terpenoid that is sparingly soluble

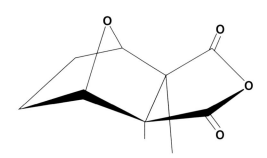

Figure 14.1
The molecular structure of cantharidin.

in water and most polar organic solvents but dissolves in oils. The crystals of cantharidins are almost colorless and odorless, and tend to be water insoluble. They are slightly soluble in alcohols and soluble in acetone at 1 : 40 dilutions. These solubility properties are important in determining the best way to mix cantharidin. Ever since Robiquet[3] initially isolated cantharidins in crystalline form, many experiments were performed in an attempt to synthesize structurally related compounds. The structural simplicity of cantharidins (Figure 14.1), and its powerful physiologic effects, elicited extreme curiosity within the scientific community.

Insects producing cantharidins are beetles belonging to the order Coleoptera, family Meloidae, and are well known as 'blister beetle'.[1,2] The dried and powdered blister beetle is called cantharides. The most well-recognized beetles are *Cantharis vesicatoria* or 'Spanish fly' which resides in southern Europe. There are approximately 1500 different species of cantharidin-yielding beetles, with a few located in the USA. The blood, soft tissues, and ovaries of these blister beetle have the highest concentration of cantharidin.[2] The average cantharidin content for the different species of beetles ranges form 2.6 to 4.3 parts per thousand (ppt).

Studies done by Bodenstein[7] showed that the South African beetle *Mylabridae* might have one of the highest averages of 11 ppt.

The effects of cantharidin on normal skin include acantholysis and death of the epidermal cells.[6] There is an intact basal layer with minimal reaction in the dermis, which results in the absence of scarring. In fact, acantholysis occurs mostly in the upper half of the wart, producing a mid-epidermal blister. It is the physical disruption of the epidermal cells that ultimately leads to the curative action of warts.

The mode of action of cantharidin is currently under investigation; however, many scientists after Unna showed evidence that acantholysis was the result of protease activation.[8] It was also widely accepted that cantharidins poisoned mitochondria and caused resultant changes in the cell membrane, epidermal cell dyscohesion, and subsequent acantholysis.[9] Stoughton[10] first showed that cantharidin acts by altering a cutaneous enzyme or enzyme system. Specifically, he believed that cantharidin-induced acantholysis was caused by activation of a disulfide-splitting enzyme present but hidden in the normal skin. Weakley and Einbinder[11] in 1961 proposed that acantholysis was mediated by the glutathione reductase enzyme. Yell et al[12] described these changes occurring as a result of the loss of extracellular glycosylated protein molecules, possibly caused by proteolysis or the modification and internalization of extracellular domains. They hypothesized that the changes were analogous to those seen in Darier's and Hailey–Hailey diseases. Although the mechanism of acantholysis resulting from cantharidins is still controversial, there is general agreement that there is a modification of certain proteins which leads to disruption of the intercellular bridges, ultimately resulting in the blistering properties.

CLINICAL STUDIES

In view of the known blistering effect on the skin of cantharidins, it was proposed that it would be an ideal destructive modality in the treatment of warts. The first clinical studies using cantharidins in the treatment of warts were performed in 1957 by Epstein and Kligman.[6] For topical treatments, cantharidin was prepared as a 0.7% solution in equal parts acetone and flexible collodion. The cantharidin was first dissolved in acetone and the solution was kept in a tightly stoppered bottle. Evaporation was minimal; however, the solution may be reconstituted by adding acetone and ether (50 : 50). A drop of the solution was rubbed over the wart. The lesion was occluded with plastic adhesive tape that was placed on the wart. They then covered the preparation with Band-Aid or gauze dressings. The dressing was left in place for 7–10 days. Subsequently, the altered skin was débrided with a knife during the next visit to the surgery. Reapplication of the preparation was made on a weekly basis after evaluation of the persistence of the wart. The results of this study showed that, of 113 warts in 61 patients, the cure rate approached 80% for common, plantar, and periungual warts. They claimed that cantharidins were no more effective than other destructive techniques; however, their usefulness rested in their simplicity of application and lack of residual scarring.

Panzwar[13] showed in 1961 that the same preparation of cantharidin was also useful when the wart was occluded with 40% salicylic acid plaster. This article initiated the synergistic use of multiple chemotherapeutic modalities in the successful treatment of warts.

During 1977, Rosenberg et al[14] published an article advocating the weekly use of cantharidins at home. The cantharidin was supplied as a 0.7% solution in acetone and flexible collodion in 2.5 ml applicator bottles for the patient's ease of application. They used a food color and omitted the use of occlusive tape to facilitate the process for the patient. They treated a total of 336 hand warts in 100 patients. Of these 336, 150 were common and 178 were subungual and paronychial warts. The treatment removed 112 of 178 (63%) subungual or paronychial warts and 103 of 158 (65%) common warts. They showed that home treatment with 0.7% cantharidin was a safe, easy, and effective method for the treatment of warts.

In 1984, Coskey published an article about the treatment of plantar warts in children with a combination of salicylic–podophyllin and cantharidin solution.[13] After initially débriding the wart with a single-edge razor blade, a preparation containing 30% salicylic acid, 5% podophyllin, 1% cantharidin, and 0.5% penederm in a film-forming base was applied to the wart, and the area was occluded with a Band-Aid. This preparation was left in place for 24 hours. The patient was seen 1 week later; the area was débrided, and silver nitrate was applied to the base of the débrided area. The results showed a cure rate of 81%. Cantharidin, podophyllin, and salicylic components were previously used individually to treat warts, but this was the first study to treat warts with a combination of these compounds, and this combination is still widely used.

In 1991, Goldfarb et al[15] reviewed the literature and confirmed that cantharidin was very successful in the removal of warts when compared with other available modalities. One of the most recent published articles by Robson et al[16] compared conventional therapy (liquid nitrogen cryotherapy or cantharidin agents) and pulsed dye laser. Of the 20 patients in the conventional therapy group, 18 received exclusively cryotherapy, one received exclusively cantharidin, and one received a combination of cryotherapy and cantharidin in sequence. The results showed a complete response rate of 70% in patients treated with conventional therapy and 65% in pulse dye laser-treated patients. This is similar to the success rate of cantharidin therapy reported previously.

In summary, over the last five decades, multiple clinical studies have demonstrated that cantharidin therapy can be successful in removing warts.[6,13,14,16,17] These include well-designed cohort or case-control analytic studies.[15–17] The results of such studies have shown an average cure rate of 80%.[18]

Using our Modified Evidence-based Medicine System (see Chapter 19), the evidence presented is rated only level III until longer randomized clinical trials are performed. Of course, the special advantages of this treatment including its ease of application, cost-efficiency, and absence of scarring will ensure the widespread use of this modality pending new evidence.

FAVORED TREATMENT METHODOLOGY

Cantharidins can be used as a single preparation or in combination with other chemotherapeutic modalities, including salicylic acid and/or podophyllin.

Many modifications of Epstein and Kligman's methods have been attempted; however, there have not been drastic changes in the administration of cantharidin in the treatment of warts.[6]

Whether using cantharidin prepared as a 0.7% solution in equal parts of acetone and flexible collodion, or as a combination of cantharidin, salicylic acid, and podophyllin in several different concentrations (Cantharone, Cantharone Plus, or Verr-Canth), there are minor differences in the methodology (Table 14.1). The cantharidin solution should be applied to the wart with the wooden end of a cotton-tipped applicator and occluded with tape (Blenderm) for 24 hours.[19] With the combination therapy, the wart is occluded for a shorter duration of 2 hours. The remaining procedure is the same for each cantharidin mixture and includes direct removal of occlusive tape or soaking it off with water. The area

Table 14.1 Cantharidin treatment methodology

Medication	Occlusion time (h)
Cantharidin 0.7% with acetone	24
Cantharone (cantharidin collodion 0.7%)	6
Cantharone Plus (salicyclic acid 30%, podophyllin resin 5% and cantharidin 1%)	2

is adequately washed with a mild soap. If the blisters become tense and painful, they should be drained with a blade or sterile needle. Treatment should be repeated weekly after thorough débridement of the dead tissue. The average number of treatments needed to eradicate the warts is usually one to five; however, some patients may not respond to this chemotherapeutic treatment.

There are many advantages and disadvantages in the use of cantharidin therapy[6,19] (Table 14.2). The advantages of cantharidins include the assurance of compliance in treatment in the surgery. There is also little pain with the application of topical treatments. The major disadvantages include possible pain 12–24 hours after application, tense blister formation, and the requirement of multiple visits to the surgery for repeated treatments. There have also been changes in the Food and Drug Administration (FDA) status of cantharidin that require that the product be produced from ingredients at local pharmacies.

Table 14.2 Adverse effects of topical cantharidins on skin

Local reactions:
 Erythema
 Tingling
 Itching
 Burning
 Tenderness
 Pain
 Aseptic necrosis of wart
 Formation of ring wart around treatment site
Systemic reactions:
 Lymphangitis
 Urgency
 Hematuria
 Tachycardia
 Profuse sweating
 Pain: distal end of penis
 Dysuria
 Oliguria

ADVERSE EFFECTS

The adverse effects of these drugs are generally mild and most often include local reactions at the application site; however, rare systemic reactions have been published (Table 14.3). The main adverse effects of topical cantharidins include local reactions such as pain, tenderness, and discomfort.[6] Other articles have reported local reactions including edema, erythema, and lymphangitis manifested as red streaks running proximally on the legs and forearms.[20] These changes have been refuted and attributed to aseptic necrosis of the wart.[21]

Table 14.3 Toxicological effects of cantharidins (oral ingestion)

Mouth

Burning of lips, mouth and pharynx
Ulcerations/excoriations of lip and buccal mucosa
Swollen tongue

Gastrointestinal

Nausea
Vomiting
Diarrhoea
Midline abdominal pain
Abdominal tenderness
Hematemesis

Genitourinary

Frequency, dysuria, hematuria
Flank pain
Oliguria
Acute tubular necrosis
Priapism
Renal failure

Cardiac

Sinus tachycardia
Arrhythmias (ventricular fibrillation, asystole)
Multiple punctate hemorrhages in pericardium/subendocardium

Hematologic

Leukocytosis
Pseudopolycythemia

Neurologic

Dilated pupils with non-reactive to light
Numbness of hands and feet
'Glove and stocking' type peripheral neuropathy
Diminished deep tendon reflexes
Bilateral lower motor neuron lesions

Pulmonary

Pulmonary edema
Coma
Death

Summarized from Ellenhorn et al.[1]

Another common adverse reaction after application of cantharidin includes the formation of a ring ('donut') wart. The study done by Rosenberg et al[14] showed that, out of 100 patients treated for a total of 336 hand warts, none of the patients experienced pain, blistering, or other side effects. A single patient, however, developed a 'fairy ring of tiny satellite warts' on the palms after the original warts were eradicated. The mechanism of ring wart formation includes the eradication of the central portion of the lesion. After multiple treatments, the periphery of the wart contains viral particles which proliferate and produce a circumferential area of wart. Treatment of the ring wart is by reapplication of cantharidin, but a more popular approach includes the use of cryotherapy.

Other disadvantages of cantharidin therapy include the possible requirement of multiple visits to the surgery. This is not consistent throughout the entire population treated; however, it is generally accepted that it may require one to five treatments for the eradication of viral warts

Adverse reactions after application of a toxic quantity of cantharidin to the skin results in inflammation to blistering within 4–5 hours to death within 12 hours.[2] Skin lesions caused by toxic doses should be cleansed with acetone, ether, fatty soap, or alcohol. These agents dissolve and dilute the cantharidin. The lesion should be cleansed repeatedly with soap and water. Calamine lotion containing a steroid may be useful. Treatment is mostly symptomatic and supportive.

Cantharidins taken orally are responsible for acute poisoning and include toxicity for many organ systems (Table 14.4). Patients have survived after ingestion of 75 mg, 175 mg, and 20 mg.[1] Fatal doses have varied between 10 mg and 65 mg. Toxic levels of this drug had disastrous effects on multiple organ systems, including abdominal pain, nausea, vomiting, hematuria, oliguria, renal failure, sinus tachycardia, ventricular fibrillation, asystole, peripheral neuropathy, pulmonary edema, coma, and even death.

Table 14.4 Patient education sheet

What are cantharidins?
Cantharidin is a blistering agent that causes the superficial layer of the epidermis containing the wart and human papillomavirus (HPV) virions to blister. The blister causes sloughing of tissue which destroys the wart physically. The main advantage of this particular treatment modality is that it does not involve cutting that would leave a scar, and there is a minimal amount of pain. It is important to understand that a single treatment may cure the wart; however, multiple treatments may be required. The treatment approaches an 80% cure rate and there is no guarantee that this topical pharmacologic treatment will work for you. Other methods may be used if this one proves unsuccessful.

Before treatment
- The wart and the surrounding area are evaluated
- Education about the nature of the disease is provided and the risks and benefits of cantharidin therapy are discussed
- The area of the wart is cleaned with alcohol prep

During treatment
- The doctor will apply the medicine to the warts during the visit to the surgery
- You will feel and cold surface as the solution is put on to the wart with a wooden applicator
- An occlusive tape and then a Band-Aid will be put on the surface which must stay on for 2 hours
- Tell your doctor about any changes associated with the administration of the topical medication at the local site or other generalized symptoms

After treatment
- At the end of the 2–hour period, remove the occlusive tape and Band-Aid and wash the medicine off with soap and water (just rinsing is not good enough)
- If you have difficulty removing the tape, you may soak the areas in warm, soapy water first
- Later in the day, you will notice that you have redness, pain or a blister (sometimes all three may occur at once)
- If blister causes pain, you may sterilize a needle and drain the blister; otherwise, nothing needs to be done
- Call the physician if you have any problems with a tense or painful blister
- May need to come back to the physician's surgery for the wound to be débrided weekly
- Do not be upset if the warts do not completely disappear after a single administration; as we never know how deep a wart is, multiple applications may be required, especially if the wart is located in the palms and soles; bleeding into the blister may occur giving them a black color
- Return to your doctor if warts persist, new lesions occur, or if 'ring-like' lesions develop at the site of a previous treatment.

COST–BENEFIT CONSIDERATIONS

The cost of a bottle of cantharidin, either as cantharidin collodion or as a mixture with salicylic acid and podophyllin, on average, is approximately $US40 for a 7.5-ml bottle. A single bottle can be used to treat hundreds of viral warts. The actual cost to the patient of using cantharidin therapy is made up of the physician visit and the procedure of Cantharone application. The cost of the application of Cantharone Plus varies according to the physician and insurance company, but ranges from approximately $US50–60 for a single wart to $US10–15 each for 2–14 treated warts; 15 or more treated warts cost a set fee of approximately $US250, e.g. if a new patient has two warts that need to be removed, and assuming the average number of treatments required is usually two, then the total cost would be $US118. The indirect costs include any post-treatment wound care and pain medication, which are rare and minimal. Cantharidin therapy is associated with a very high success rate, with relatively low recurrence, similar to that of other modalities; however, cantharidins are much cheaper to administer and therefore both the direct and indirect costs are lower than most other treatment options. In conclusion, cantharidin therapy is a very effective and cost-efficient method of eliminating warts.

CASE REPORTS

Case 1

The patient is a 17-year-old man who presented for evaluation of multiple warts on his feet. Physical examinations revealed seven warts, three on the right foot and four on the left, concentrated on the ball of the foot. All of the lesions were less than 3.0 mm in diame-

ter. The patient was treated with Cantharone Plus for 2 hours. Follow-up during the subsequent week revealed pain in the last few days such that the patient had not been able to go to school. On physical examination, there were multiple large blisters in the previously treated areas (Figure 14.2a). The lesion was unroofed and the patient was treated again with Cantharone for 6 hours on the following day. At 1-week follow-up, there was excellent improvement in the patient's warts (Figure 14.2b). There was just a hint of wart remaining in a few areas on both feet after paring. The lesion was treated again with Cantharone for 6 hours. After another 2-weeks of follow-up there was resolution of the warts on both feet, with a pinpoint wart on the left big toe. The lesion was treated again with Cantharone for 6 hours. During a follow-up 2 weeks later, there was complete clearance of all the warts. The patient has not had any recurrence since.

Case 2

An 11-year-old boy presented with a year's history of warts on his right and left hands. This was his initial visit and the warts had not been previously treated. Physical examinations revealed a dozen 2.0- to 6.0-mm warts on his right and left hands. Education about the nature of the disease was provided to the patient and guardian, and the risks and benefits of cantharidin therapy were discussed. Cantharidin therapy was initiated using a 0.7% cantharidin solution (Cantharone Plus) applied for 2 hours. Within 1 week, the patient showed excellent improvement, with only four warts left on each hand. After another week of treatment, all but one wart on the third right finger were eradicated. One month subsequent to weekly therapy with cantharidin, the patient presented with a recurrent wart on his right thumb, where it made a large donut lesion 1.3 cm in diameter (Figure 14.3). The lesion was treated with multiple

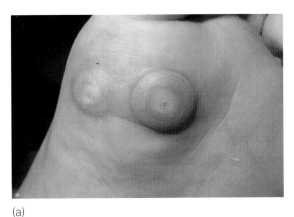
(a)

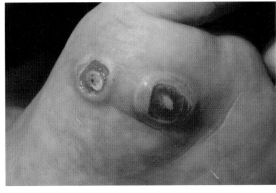
(b)

Figure 14.2
(a) These tender blisters occurred overlying two plantar warts 1 day after application of cantharidin/podophyllin/salicylic acid (Cantharone Plus) under occlusion for 2 hours. (b) The blister was unroofed with a no. 15 blade, resulting in immediate relief of pain and demonstrating persistent wart at the base of the blister, which required additional treatment.

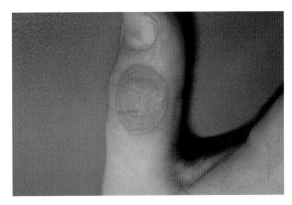

Figure 14.3
The feared ring wart or 'donut' wart which recurred 1 month after cantharidin treatment of a wart on the right thumb, which initially appeared to have cleared.

applications of liquid nitrogen and subsequently disappeared. The patient has not had any recurrence since the time of presentation.

REFERENCES

1. Ellenhorn JE, Schonwald S, Ordog G, Wasserberger J. *Ellenhorn's Medical Toxicology. Diagnosis and Treatment of Human Poisoning*, 2nd edn. Baltimore: Williams & Wilkins, 1997: 1813–15.
2. Till JS, Majmuder BN. Cantharidin poisoning. *South Med J* 1981; **74**: 444–7.
3. Robiquet M. *Ann Chim* 1810; **76**: 302–7.
4. Unna, PG. *The Histopathology of the Diseases of the Skin*, translated by Norman Walker. Edinburgh: WF Clay, 1896: 98.
5. Vichower A, Cohen I. Mechanism of action of aphrodisiacs and other irritant drugs. *Am J Pharmacol* 1938; **110**: 226.
6. Epstein WL, Kligman AM. Treatment of warts with cantharidin. *Arch Dermatol* 1958; **77**: 508–11
7. Bodenstein JC. Determination of cantharidin in beetles and native medicines. *Analyst* 1943; **68**: 238.

8. Pierard-Franchimont C, Pierard GE. Cantharidin-induced acantholysis. *Am J Dermatopathol* 1988; **5**: 419–23

9. Swinyard EA, Pathak MA. Locally acting drugs. Surface-acting drugs. In: Gilman AG, Goodman LS, Gilman A, eds. *Goodman and Gilman's Pharmacologic Basis of Therapeutics*, 6th edn. New York: Macmillan, 1980.

10. Stoughton RB, Novack N. Disruption of epithelial bridges by disulfide splitting agents. *J Invest Dermatol* 1956; **16**: 127.

11. Weakley DR, Eikenbinder JM. The mechanics of cantharidin acantholysis. *J Invest Dermatol* 1962; 39–45.

12. Yell JA, Burge SM, Dean D. Cantharidin-induced acantholysis: adhesion molecules, protease proteins. *Br J Dermatol* 1994; **2**: 148–57.

13. Panzwer HM. Cantharidin – a useful agent in the local treatment of warts. *J Germantown Hosp* 1961; **2**: 82–6.

14. Rosenberg EW, Amonette RA, Gardner JH. Cantharidin treatment of warts at home (letter to the editor). *Arch Dermatol* 1977; **113**: 1134.

15. Goldfarb MT, Gupta AK, Gupta MA, Sawchuk WS. Office therapy for human papillomavirus infection in nongenital sites. *Dermatol Clin* 1991; **9**: 287–96.

16. Robson KJ, Cunningham NM, Kruzan KL et al. Pulsed-dye laser versus conventional therapy in the treatment of warts: A prospective randomized trial. *J Am Acad Dermatol* 2000; **43**: 275–80.

17. Coskey JR. Treatment of plantar warts in children with a salicylic acid–podophyllin–cantharidin product. *Pediatric Dermatology*.

18. Sterling JC, Handfield-Jones S, Hudson PM. Guidelines for the management of cutaneous warts. *Br J Dermatol* 2001; **144**: 4–10.

19. Miller DM, Brodell RT. Human papillomavirus infection: treatment options for warts. *Am Family Physic* 1996; **53**: 135–43.

20. Dilaimy M. Lymphangitis caused by cantharidin (letter to the editor). *Arch Dermatol* 1975; **111**: 1073.

21. Roth HL. Aseptic necrosis of warts instead of lmphangitis (letter to the editor). *Arch Dermatol* 1976; **112**: 1035.

15 Contact immunotherapy in the treatment of viral warts

Zulma I Toledo and Robert T Brodell

Historical aspects • Basic science • Clinical evidence • Adverse effects • Other agents • Cost comparison between agents • Case report • References

Human papillomavirus (HPV) is a highly resilient, non-enveloped, double-stranded DNA virus that is tropic for epithelial cells. There have been more than 70 genotypically distinct HPV types identified. The large number of HPV types poses a technical problem in devising vaccines. Alternative methods of inducing an immune response include the use of intralesional skin test antigens (see Chapter 17), topical imiquimod (see Chapter 6), intralesional interferon (see Chapter 12), and contact immunotherapy. All of these methods hold the promise of efficacy, lower risk of recurrence, and an absence of scarring. For now, these agents remain *alternative* treatments for warts resistant to first-line agents.

HISTORICAL ASPECTS

In 1969, Klein[1] reported 'Dinitrochlorobenzene is a potent stimulator of cutaneous T-cell sensitivity'. He showed that dinitrochlorobenzene (DNCB) could induce specific cell-mediated immunity, resulting in complete resolution of basal cell carcinoma and squamous cell carcinoma. Klein[1] felt that DNCB elicited a much stronger immune response on neoplastic tissue than on adjacent normal tissue.

Verrucae are a form of rapidly proliferating tissue resulting from viral infection and are analogous in many ways to neoplastic tissue.

In 1973, both Lewis[2] and Greenberg et al[3] reported the use of DNCB contact immunotherapy for resistant warts. There were at least five additional reports on the use of DNCB published between 1973 and 1984. Squaric acid dibutylester (SABDE) and diphenylcyclopropenone (DPCP) immunotherapy for warts was reported in 1974. Although further studies in the 1980s supported the use of these agents, there have been no additional studies since the late 1980s.

BASIC SCIENCE

The process of contact immunotherapy requires a substance that can reliably induce type IV hypersensitivity. Ideally, this substance should be readily available and able to sensitize at least 95% of normal individuals. It should be both chemically stable and economical. Even more importantly, it should have minimal adverse effects. Finally, the substance should be rare in the environment because induction of allergic contact dermatitis in sensitized individuals could cause significant morbidity.

Allergic contact dermatitis is the prototype of delayed hypersensitivity reaction (type IV hypersensitivity). The process of delayed hypersensitivity has two phases: the induction phase and the elicitation phase. The induction phase is the period from the initial contact with a chemical until lymphocytes have been 'educated' to respond to that particular chemical. The elicitation phase is the period from re-exposure to the chemical in a sensitized individual to the appearance of dermatitis.

In a simplistic view of the induction phase there are three main players: the allergen, the Langerhans' cell, and the T lymphocyte. Not all chemicals induce an allergic reaction. In addition, one chemical will not sensitize everyone. Sensitization depends not only on the chemical, but also on the nature of the exposure and the genetic susceptibility and non-genetic idiosyncrasies of the person. Certain chemicals routinely produce sensitization in most patients, e.g. DNCB sensitizes about 97% of the white population after appropriate contact. On the other hand, lanolin rarely induces allergic contact dermatitis despite the almost universal and continual exposure to human skin in hand creams and cosmetics. Most allergenic chemicals are small, reactive, lipid-soluble chemicals that easily penetrate the skin; they are called haptens, because these chemicals are not allergens by themselves.

For the immune system to react, the hapten is presented to it by a carrier protein on the surface of Langerhans' cells. Langerhans' cells lie in the epidermis and, once the haptens diffuse down from the skin's surface and bind to the dendritic processes of the Langerhans' cells, the 'unit' migrates into the dermis. T lymphocytes identify the hapten–carrier complex and initiate the events that lead to induction of allergic contact dermatitis. The initiation process usually requires Langerhans' cells to carry antigen to regional lymph nodes. Here they present antigen to those T lymphocytes that have been genetically programmed to interact with a particular antigen. The antigen-stimulated lymphocytes enlarge and can then be recognized histologically as immunoblasts. These immunoblasts divide and, although some clones travel to skin sites to serve as effector cells, others remain in nodes or other sites and serve as memory cells to evoke skin reactions with subsequent contact with allergens – even years later. (Memory cells are long lived compared with effector cells.)

Persistence of allergen at a skin site or reintroduction of the same allergen at other skin sites initiates the elicitation phase, producing the inflammatory reaction of allergic contact dermatitis. In this phase, effector lymphocytes travel to the skin, where they contact the processed allergen (the hapten and its carrier protein on the surface of the Langerhans' cells). Even though the elicitation reactions recapitulate induction reactions with respect to capturing, processing, and presenting antigens to the appropriate lymphocytes, the objective of the immune system is now to elicit inflammation in order to destroy the antigen.[4]

How is this process translated into a therapeutic modality for extragenital cutaneous warts? There are several theories – none of which has been proved with certainty. In the first scenario a soluble antigen painted on the surface of a wart induces a type IV hypersensitivity reaction. This inflammation damages virally infected cells, which are innocent bystanders. This is a non-wart-antigen-specific destructive effect.[5]

A second theory hypothesizes that the applied substance acts as a hapten attaching to wart proteins and then induces a *specific* immune reaction to wart antigen. This was the explanation originally proposed for the effect of DNCB on malignant tumors.[1] There is conflicting evidence relating to this theory. Anecdotal evidence is often provided to support this theory. In one case, DNCB was used to induce allergic contact hypersensitivity. There was complete clearing of all verrucae. New verrucae developed about 6 months later. Over a 3-week period the new verrucae spontaneously became inflamed and regressed without further DNCB application. Concurrently one of the primary DNCB sensitization sites on the patient's arm also reacted. This suggests that DNCB and wart viral antigen cross-react. Similarly, other current treatment modalities such as cryotherapy may be successful, partly because they indirectly induce cell-mediated immunity to wart antigens by releasing immature viral particles from disrupted epithelium, thus exposing them to antigen-processing cells.[5]

Anecdotal evidence provided by other experts opposes these concepts. In their experience it was unusual for warts to resolve in areas not actively treated. This makes actions that are wart-antigen-specific and T-cell cytotoxic an unlikely primary mechanism. In addition, as reinfection commonly occurs, long-lasting immunity typical of antigen-specific cell-mediated immunity does not appear to be conferred by therapy.[6]

The importance of humoral immunity in contact immunotherapy is less controversial.[7] Complement-binding wart virus antibodies increase from 15% before contact immunotherapy with DNCB to 48% afterwards. Natural killer cells, macrophages, and granulocytes are effector cells for antibody-dependent cell-mediated cytotoxicity. These effector cells bind and lyse antibody-bearing target cells.[6] In addition, lymphocytes produce lymphokines (interleukin-2 and interferon) that potentiate the process. These cells may also decrease suppressive influences that inhibit the host reaction to warts.[5]

In summary, the exact mechanism of wart destruction after contact immunotherapy may involve: (1) destruction that is non-wart antigen specific (wart destroyed as an innocent bystander),[5] (2) wart-antigen-specific destruction,[1] (3) activation of humoral factor leading to destruction,[6] or (4) combinations of each of these mechanisms.

CLINICAL EVIDENCE

The clinical evidence available to support the use of DNCB as a treatment for recurrent or recalcitrant non-genital warts is presented in Table 15.1. The percentage of patients cleared with applications of DNCB was between 69% and 91%, and recurrence rates were generally low. Some variations among these studies lie in the concentrations of DNCB used, vehicles, frequency of treatments, patient-applied treatments vs surgery/physician-instituted therapy, and length of therapy. Decisions about the frequency of application of these contact agents are rooted in basic science. Langerhans' cells, which are thought to be necessary for antigen processing, quickly disappear at the site of inflammatory response. Therefore, the daily application used in some studies may be no more effective than bi-weekly treatments.[5] Almost invariably, DNCB was used in conjunction with subsequent occlusive bandages. This is important to keep the antigen from contacting areas of normal skin that would provoke an unnecessary allergic contact dermatitis on normal skin.

All these studies suggest that therapy with DNCB clears warts faster than expected in view of the natural history of these lesions. The best evidence about the natural history of warts suggests that one-third of untreated warts resolve spontaneously in 6 months and two-thirds in 2 years.[5] However, only 40% of patients had complete resolution of warts in 2 years during this study. Furthermore, warts that have proved resistant to cryotherapy or other conventional treatments might be expected to have even less favorable rates of spontaneous regression.

No double-masked studies with DNCB have been performed, because the inflammation response is readily apparent and would be distinguishable from a placebo control by both the patient and the clinical researcher. The use of an agent such as croton oil might offer a solution to this problem. It would prove inter-

Table 15.1 Dinitrochlorobenzene (DNCB)

Author	Type of study	No. of patients	Percentage cleared	Special notes
Lewis[2]	Case reports	77	91	Daily applications of DNCB in Aquaphor under Telfa occlusion with concurrent use of salicylic acid plasters
Greenberg et al[3]	Case–control study	N/A	N/A	Performed biopsy examination on all patients in order to investigate histology Effects of biopsy examination are unknown
Dunagis and Millikan[5]	Case reports	24	87	Applied 400 µg of DNCB in acetone at 2- to 3-week intervals covered with non-occlusive gauze
Eriksen[7]	Case–control study	43	80	Used sufficient DNCB in acetone or dimethyl sulfoxide to maintain type IV allergic reaction
Goiham and Yahr[8]	Case reports	40	83	Used variable concentrations of DNCB (0.1% most frequently) Patients self-applied therapy. (most application < 400 µg)
Buckner and Price[9]	Case reports	35	69	Used challenge doses of 0.1% DNCB in soft paraffin applied by patients at unspecified intervals
Nater et al[10]	Case–control study	13	85	Used 2% solution of DNCB
Claudy and Roche[11]	Case reports	22	81	Used sufficient concentrations to produce an allergic reaction

esting to assess the effectiveness of inflammation from irritation caused by croton oil, when compared with an allergic contact dermatitis induced by contact immunotherapy.

ADVERSE EFFECTS

DNCB immunotherapy is associated with significant side effects. Patients remain allergic for an extended period of time, and perhaps forever. Therefore, they are susceptible to allergic contact dermatitis on re-exposure. Fortunately, DNCB is rarely encountered outside the laboratory. Of course, patients may spread the chemical from the site of application to normal skin, thus acquiring an unanticipated contact dermatitis. Lewis[2] reported one patient who developed generalized autosensitization. Cross-reactivity between chloramphenicol and DNCB has been hypothesized, but studies in guinea-pigs and humans have shown no evidence of cross-reaction.[12] By far the most disconcerting potential of DNCB is the possibility that it may be a carcinogen.

The reports of DNCB as a mutagen and carcinogen are based on microbial studies that use the Ames' method, which is a useful and relatively inexpensive, short-term, in vitro screening test for mutagenicity.[13,14] However, not all Ames' tests with DNCB are in accordance. Furthermore, in contrast to the in vitro test documenting mutagenicity, in vivo studies have not yet revealed any carcinogenic activity of DNCB. However, the DNCB precursor mononitrochlorobenzenes show definite carcinogenicity. Both forms of these benzenes induced a significant increase in vascular, liver, and other multiple tumors in male and female mice and rats.[15] The presence of either of these contaminants would allow unnecessary exposure of patients to a carcinogenic substance.[13] Even small amounts of contaminants might be significant because up to 65% of topical DNCB is absorbed when acetone is used as a vehicle. One study found no mononitrochlorobenzene contamination of DNCB.[13]

Taking into consideration all the above, we believe that the use of DNCB for benign skin diseases should be abandoned, especially in light of new alternative contact allergens such as SABDE and diphencypropene (DCP) which are discussed later. This is based on the following factors:

1. The correlation between mutagenicity in the Ames' test and carcinogenicity in mammals is up to 90%.
2. DNCB has been shown to cause cell transformation in cultured mammalian cells.
3. Strobel and Rohrborn[12,16] tested DNCB when added to a standardized cell line of baby Syrian hamster kidney cells; they noted a dose-dependent increase of clones of transformed cells that far exceeded the spontaneous frequency in the absence of DNCB. These results were obtained with and without metabolic activation by rat liver S9 fraction. Although these experiments still do not provide proof of carcinogenicity in humans, it should be realized that this assay is approximately 90% accurate in discriminating carcinogens and non-carcinogens.
4. Studies from Black[17] also showed that DNCB by itself is mutagenic in the bacterial plate incorporation assay.
5. It should be mentioned that a fluoro-derivative of DNCB, 1-fluoro-2,4-dinitrobenzene, has been shown to be a potent tumor-promoting agent in mice treated with 7,12-dimethylbenzen[a]anthracene. The structure of DNCB is such that it is likely to behave in the same way, in addition to its mutagenic potential.[14]

OTHER AGENTS

SABDE is another agent that can be used to treat warts by inducing a type IV hypersensitivity reaction. It sensitizes at least 95% of normal individuals and is not found in normal human environments. It is chemically stable and inexpensive to produce. There is no evidence of mutagenicity in the Ames' test.

Table 15.2 presents the clinical evidence available to support the use of SABDE as a contact immunotherapy agent to treat warts. One study[18] found it to be ineffective in the treatment of warts. The other studies,[19–21] including the largest study performed more recently, found SABDE to be effective, with clinical resolution in 86% of patients and few side effects.[21]

Treatment with SABDE is well tolerated by patients. The use of SABDE is a logical choice for recalcitrant warts, especially in younger patients who do not tolerate painful destructive procedures such as cryotherapy.[20]

Other agents used to induce contact immunotherapy for treatment to resistant warts have emerged, probably as a result of the concerns over the potential carcinogenicity of the most popular agent DNCB. Some of these agents are Rhus antigen, DCP, and

Table 15.2 Squaric acid dibutylester (SABDE)

Author	Type of study	No. of patients	Percentage cleared	Special notes
Claudy and Roche[18]	Case–control study	18	10	They concluded that SABDE was ineffective Used 11 weeks of weekly treatment with poor cure rate Raised question of age-dependent contact immunotherapy, with higher cure rates noted in patients younger than 15
Ijima and Otsuka[19]	Case reports	20	60	Achieved wart regression within 3 months with an average of six treatments
Lee and Mallory[20]	Case reports		69	Achieved complete regression within 12 months with a mean of 5.9 treatments Used higher SABDE concentration at less frequent intervals, but reported a higher incidence of severe contact dermatitis Reported hypopigmentation at sites of SABDE application
Micali et al[21]	Case–control study	443	86	Observed that periungual and subungual warts had the longest resolution time, suggesting that location of warts may be a critical issue Noted patients treated with SABDE for alopecia areata had resolution of the warts on the back of their hands Treatment had no systemic effects and treatments were well tolerated

DPCP. These agents have been used with good results and few side effects. These studies are summarized in Table 15.3.

Although these studies were flawed in many ways (only partially prospective, lacking defined long-term follow-up evidence), a 70–88% remission rate within 5–14 months is comparable or better than reports from open-label studies of other therapies.

Also of note, a precursor of DCP, dibenzyldibromoketone, is found to be mutagenic by the Ames' assay. Therefore, the production of DCP requires appropriate purification because this chemical lacks patent protection, and there is little financial incentive for product development.[23]

Rhus antigen lacks research appeal, most probably because it is easily contacted in human environments.[6] According to our Modified Evidence-based Medicine System (Chapter 19), contact immunotherapy agents are supported by level III evidence. DNCB

Table 15.3 Other agents

Author	Type of study	No. of patients	Percentage cleared	Special notes
Upitis[22]	Retrospective study	154	88	Began treatment with 1% DPCP over 6 months, increasing DPCP strength up to 4% to maintain clinical response with minimal side effects Side effects (pruritus, local blistering and eczematous reactions) were well tolerated and expected
Buckley et al[23]	Case reports	60	88	Applied DCP (0.01–6.0%) in the surgery to pared warts at 1- to 4-week interval; additional paring and keratolytics were encouraged Side effects included localized and generalized vesicular dermatitis and lymphadenopathy in 57% of patients

Table 15.4 Patient education sheet

What is contact immunotherapy as a treatment against warts?
It is a process by which your own body is stimulated to reject your warts. Your dermatologist applies a substance on your skin that stimulates your own immune system to attack and destroy those unsightly warts you've been trying so hard to get rid of! Your body will be mounting an allergic reaction to the warts. Contact immunotherapy is usually reserved for warts that have been resistant to other conventional surgery and home treatments available for warts. Why? Because not everything is understood about the mechanism the body uses to destroy the warts. Many unanswered questions also remain with regard to the substances used to induce the contact immunotherapy. We will refer to it as a tool available to your dermatologist in the quest to rid you of your warts.

What to expect during treatment?
As contact immunotherapy uses your body's immune system to attack your warts you can expect to experience a local reaction much like an allergy. You might experience itchiness, redness, swelling, and blistering over the tissue exposed to the substances used to induce the contact immunotherapy. This is why you must be very careful to apply the substance only over the wart area and wash your hands well after application. You must inform your doctor immediately of any expected and unexpected side effects. (As with any medical treatment, if you experience shortness of breath, intractable nausea and vomiting, syncope, generalized rashes or what may appear life-threatening attend an emergency room immediately. Contact your doctor as soon as possible thereafter.)

During therapy your doctor will need to see you frequently to assess the progress of therapy (initially weekly) and after a while he might ask you to apply the substances at home if you feel able to do so. After a while your visits will be spaced out.

Please be aware that contact immunotherapy is, as many other therapies for warts, a slow process. Resolution may take months to years and results are variable among patients. Warts may also reappear after having been totally cleared. Please call your physician with any sign of recurrence.

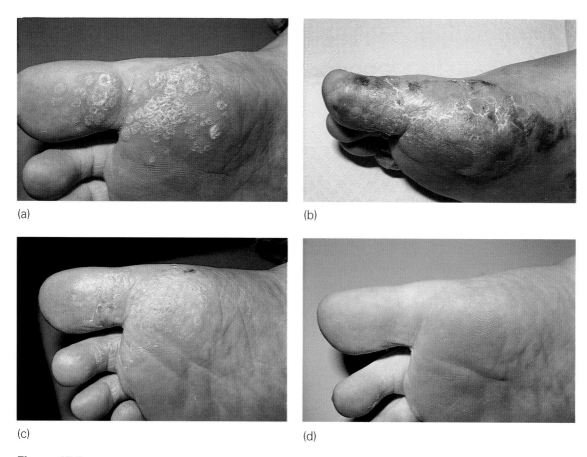

(a)

(b)

(c)

(d)

Figure 15.1

(a) Warts of 4-mm diameter are clustered in mosaic fashion broadly over the ball of the right foot and plantar surface of the big toe before starting treatment with contact immunotherapy using 1% diphenylcyclopropenone (DPCP). (b) Eight weeks after initial treatment with contact immunotherapy, the warts appear slightly thinner. Initial contact dermatitis at this site has been quieted by use of a topical steroid and alternate-day application of 1% DPCP. (c) Ten weeks after initiating contact immunotherapy, the warts are 70% improved with erythema, scaling, and edema of the treated area. (d) The warts are 95% improved 1 week after the final contact immunotherapy treatment was completed, 5 months after initial treatment. (e) Eight weeks after the final treatment with contact immunotherapy, the warts are cleared.

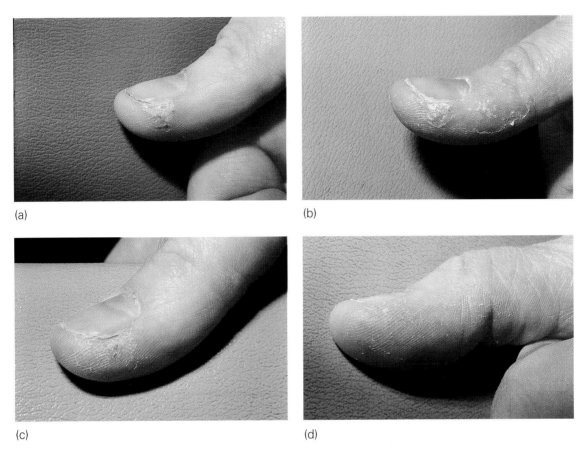

(a)

(b)

(c)

(d)

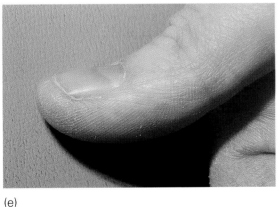

(e)

Figure 15.2

(a) A 6 × 6 mm verruca is present at the lateral nailfold of the right thumb before contact immunotherapy. (b) After 8 weeks of treatment, inflammation is present at the site of treatment on the right thumb, but little change is noted in the wart. (c) At 10 weeks after initiation of therapy with diphenylcyclopropenone (DPCP), the wart on the right thumb is 90% improved. (d) Five months after starting therapy, little wart remains. At this point, treatment was discontinued. (e) Two months after therapy was discontinued, all inflammation has subsided and no wart remains on the right thumb.

which might be rated higher based on the evidence presented, remains unrated because, as noted previously, we do not recommend its use.

COST COMPARISON BETWEEN AGENTS

Dinitrochlorobenzene is the most economical of the three agents, listed at 15 cents per gram. However, as noted above, we do not use this agent. DPCP is $US7.83 per gram and SABDE is $US37.50 per gram. The cost of an agent is also impacted by problems of stability, which can render a medicine ineffective. SABDE requires refrigeration and possibly special solvents and additives to maintain potency because of its tendency to undergo hydrolysis. DPCP must be stored in dark glass in a dark place because of its tendency to undergo photodecomposition. The main adverse effect of SABDE and DPCP is acute contact dermatitis, although dyshidrosiform hand dermatitis has been reported in two cases.

CASE REPORT

A 30-year-old woman presented for evaluation of warts on the bottom of her feet. These had been present for 12 years and had never been treated. Physical examination revealed a mosaic of warts on the plantar surface of the left ball of the foot in a 4 cm × 4 cm area and a second cluster of warts on the plantar surface of the left big toe (Figure 15.1a). A 4-mm wart was also present on the right thumb at the lateral nailfold (Figure 15.2a). After discussing all treatment options, contact immunotherapy was chosen to treat this patient because of her desire to avoid the pain associated with destructive therapies such as cryotherapy, cantharidin, and vascular lesion laser, in view of the large number of warts and large surface area affected. She was sensitized to DPCP by applying 0.1% DPCP to her left forearm, which created a papulovesicular, erythematous patch. Two weeks later DPCP was applied to her warts.

One week after this first treatment an allergic contact dermatitis was present overlying the treated wart and patch-tested site. The patient was instructed to start home application of DPCP every other night. Topical steroid cream was prescribed to help with allergic contact dermatitis as needed. The patient was seen in the doctor's surgery at 2-week intervals and the warts were noted to flatten slowly. By 6 weeks of therapy, the patient was instructed to increase home self-application of DPCP to nightly treatments. Two weeks later a brisk allergic contact dermatitis developed around her neck and arms, which was extremely pruritic. The patient was not aware of how DPCP might have been mistakenly applied to these areas. A great deal of inflammation was present at the treatment sites (Figures 15.1b and 15.2b). A 2-week rest from DPCP therapy was recommended. After this 2-week period, warts were considerably smaller in size (Figures 15.1c and 15.2c). The patient was instructed to reinstitute DPCP twice a week and increase to every other day as tolerated.

She complained of persistent itchiness around her neck and elsewhere on her body and exaggerated local inflammation on the ball of her foot with more frequent application. Therefore, at this time we reduced treatment with DPCP at home to only once a week beginning 3 months after initiation of therapy. The patient was followed up monthly and tolerated once weekly application of DPCP well. Five months after starting therapy, warts were 95% clear (Figures 15.1d and 15.2d). Treatment was discontinued. Seven months after starting therapy there was no visible remnant of the warts (Figures 15.1e and 15.2e).

REFERENCES

1. Klein E. Hypersensitivity reactions at tumor sites. *Cancer Res* 1969; **29**: 2351–62.

2. Lewis HM. Topical immunotherapy of refractory warts. *Cutis* 1973; **12**: 863–7.

3. Greenberg JH, Smith TL, Katz RM. Verruca vulgaris rejection. *Arch Dermatol* 1973; **107**: 580–2.

4. Dahl, MV. Allergic contact dermatitis. *Clin Immunodermatol*. 1996; **3**: 289–300.

5. Dunagis WG, Millikan LE. Dinitrochlorobenzene immunotherapy for verrucae resistant to standard treatment modalities. *J Am Acad Dermatol* 1982; **6**: 40–5.

6. Naylor MF, Nelder KH, Yarbrough GK et al. Contact immunotherapy of resistant warts. *J Am Acad Dermatol* 1988; **19**: 679–83.

7. Eriksen K. Treatment of the common wart by induced allergic inflammation. *Dermatologica* 1980; **160**: 161–6.

8. Goihman-Yahr M, Fernandez J, Convit J. Immunoterapia de las verrugas vulgares diseminadas con dinitrochlorobenceno. *Med Cutan Iber Lat Am* 1976; **2**: 187–94.

9. Bucker D, Price N. Immunotherapy of verrucae vulgares with dinitrochlorobenzene. *Br J Dermatol* 19??; **98**: 451–5.

10. Nater JP, Barr AJM, Bleumink E. De behandling van verrucae vulgares met 2,4-dinitrochlorobenzeen (DNCB). *Ned Tijdschr Geneeskd* 1980; **123**: 603–6.

11. Claudy AL, Roche H, Gogue Y. Traitement des verrues multiples et recidivantes par induction d'une hypersensibilité retardée. *Ann Dermatol Venereol* 19??; **107**: 551–3.

12. Storbel R, Rohborn G. Mutagenic and cell transforming activities of 1-chlor-2,4-dinitrochlorobenzene (DNCB) and squaric acid dibutylester (SABDE). *Arch Toxicol* 1980; **45**: 307–14.

13. Doubleday CW, Wilkin JK. The role of mononitrochlorobenzene as a contaminant in dinitrochlorobenzene. *J Am Acad Dermatol* 1982; **6**: 325–7.

14. Summer KH, Gogglemann W. 1-Chloro-2,4-dinitrobenzene depletes glutathione in rat skin and is mutagenic in *Salmonella typhimurium*. *Mutat Res* 1980; **77**: 91–3.

15. Weisberg EK, Russfield A, Weisburger JH. Testing of twenty one enviormental aromatic amines or derivatives for long term toxicity or carcinogenicity. *J Environ Pathol Toxicol* 1978; **2**: 235–56.

16. Kratka J, Goerz G, Vizethum W. 1-Chloro-2,4-dinitrochlorobenzene: Influence of the cytochrome P-450 system and mutagenic effects. *Arch Dermatol* 1979; **266**: 315–18.

17. Black HS, Castrow FF II, Gergius J. The mutagenicity of dinitrochlorobenzene. *Arch Dermatol* 1985; **121**: 348–9.

18. Claudy AL, Roche H. Traitement des verrues multiples et recidivantes par induction d'une hypersensibilité retardée. II etude critique de l'utilisation du dibutylester de l'acide squarique. *Ann Dermatol Venereol* 1981; **108**: 765–7.

19. Iijima S, Otsuka F. Contact immunotherapy with squaric acid dibutylester for warts. *Dermatology* 1993; **187**: 115–18.

20. Lee AN; Mallory SB. Contact immunotherapy with squaric acid dibutylester for the treatment of recalcitrant warts. *J Am Acad Dermatol* 1999; **41**: 595–9.

21. Micali G, Dall'Oglio F, Tedeshi A et al. Treatment of cutaneous warts with squaric acid dibutylester: a decade of experience. *Arch Dermatol* 2000; **136**: 557–8.

22. Upitis J. Canadian Dermatology Association. University of Alberta, Edmonton.

23. Buckley DA, Keane FM, Munn SE et al. Recalcitrant viral warts treated by diphencyprone immunotherapy. *Br J Dermatol* 1999; **141**: 292–6.

16 Cidofovir

Marla L Wirges and Sandra Marchese Johnson

Historical aspects • Basic science • Clinical studies • Adverse effects • Favored treatment methodology • Course and prognosis • Case reports • References

Cidofovir is a nucleotide analog that has activity against several DNA viruses including human papillomavirus (HPV).[1] Although only recently introduced, several reports have shown promising results for the treatment of HPV infections with both intralesional and topical cidofovir. However, randomized, placebo-controlled studies are needed to determine the exact role of cidofovir in the treatment of warts.

HISTORICAL ASPECTS

The acyclic nucleoside phosphonates represent a relatively new class of compounds that are active against a broad range of DNA viruses.[2] Cidofovir, one of the prototypes of this class of compounds, was approved by the US Food and Drug Administration in 1997 for intravenous use in the treatment of cytomegalovirus (CMV) retinitis.[3] Several case reports and a few randomized control trials have shown that cidofovir has some efficacy in the treatment of cutaneous HPV infections.

BASIC SCIENCE

Cidofovir (1-[(*S*)-3-hydroxy-2-(phosphonomethoxy)-propyl]cytosine dihydrate or HPMPC) is an

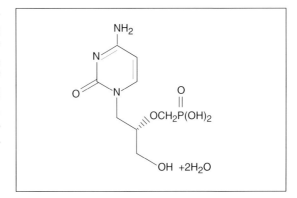

Figure 16.1
Chemical structure of cidofovir.

acyclic nucleotide analog of deoxycytidine monophosphate[4] (Figure 16.1). It has activity against a broad spectrum of DNA viruses, including Herpesviridae (Epstein–Barr virus, cytomegalovirus, varicella-zoster virus, and herpes simplex viruses 1 and 2), adenovirus, polyomavirus, and papillomavirus.[1] Cidofovir is phosphorylated into its active form, cidofovir disphosphate, by host intracellular enzymes. This differs from acyclovir, famciclovir, and ganciclovir which use virally encoded thymidine kinase for activation.[5] Cidofovir blocks viral DNA synthesis and replication by acting as a competitive inhibitor and an alternative substrate for CMV DNA polymerase[5] (Figure

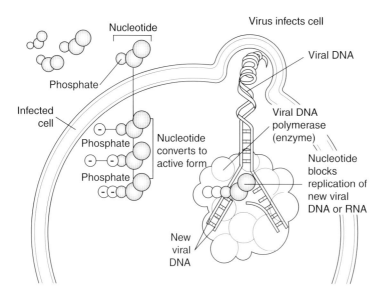

Figure 16.2
Mechanism of action of cells infected with cytomegalovirus (CMV).[14]

16.2). It inhibits viral DNA polymerase at a concentration 8- to 600-fold lower than that required to inhibit human DNA polymerase.[6]

HPV does not posses a viral DNA polymerase, so the mechanism of cell growth inhibition by cidofovir differs from that of CMV. In HPV-transformed cells treated with cidofovir, diphosphorylated HPMPC accumulates, whereas in normal cells HPMPCphosphocholine is generated.[7] This indicates that a viral factor is modulating cellular kinases and assisting in cell cycle inhibition.[7] Infected cells are trapped in the S phase of the cell cycle. Cidofovir induces DNA fragmentation in HPV16-infected cells. This is characteristic of early apoptosis and implies that cidofovir has cytotoxic effects on HPV-infected cells.[7]

CLINICAL STUDIES

Several reports have suggested that intralesional cidofovir is effective against various types of HPV infection. In 1995, Van Cutsem et al.[2] reported a case of squamous papilloma of the hypopharynx–esophagus (HPV19) successfully treated with local injections of cidofovir. Similarly, Snoeck et al[8] reported improvement of patients with severe recurrent laryngeal papillomatosis after intralesional cidofovir. Koonsaeng et al[9] completely eradicated recurrent vulvar intraepithelial neoplasia in a 43-year-women with 1% cidofovir in a Beeler base.

Recent placebo-controlled studies have shown the efficacy of topical cidofovir in the treatment of anogenital warts. Matteelli et al[10] performed a randomized, placebo-controlled, single-masked, crossover pilot study on the use of topical 1% cidofovir cream on external anogenital warts in HIV patients. Results showed that 'total wart area reduction of more often more than 50% was achieved more often with cidofovir than placebo'.[10] Recently Snoeck et al[11] published the results of a phase II, double-masked, placebo-controlled study with cidofovir gel for the treatment of condylomata accuminata; 19 patients were randomly assigned to the cidofovir group and 11 to the placebo group. Nine of the 19 (47%) patients in the active group had a complete cure and 84% had either a partial or a complete response. No patients in the placebo group had complete resolution and only two (18%) had a partial response.

Only a few additional case reports have been published using topical cidofovir to treat common warts. Zabawski et al[4] treated two patients with resistant warts with topical cidofovir. An 8-year-old girl with many resistant warts on both legs had the warts cleared with serial applications of 3% topical cidofovir. A 13-year-old with a 3-year history of warts on her fingers had her warts cleared after 10 weeks of 3% cidofovir in a Dermavan base. Davis et al[12] treated a large plantar wart (HPV66) in a 37-year-old woman with HIV with 3% cidofovir cream. By day 7 the wart had significantly regressed and by 3–4 weeks the wart had completely disappeared.

No large case series or randomized clinical trials are available therefore the strength of evidence supporting the use of cidofovir for the treatment of common warts is level IV using our Modified Evidence-based Medicine system (see Chapter 19).

ADVERSE EFFECTS

Local reactions to topical cidofovir are common and occasionally severe. Burning, pain, erythema, inflammation, and pruritus are frequently reported and may be severe enough to require termination of treatment. Erosions and ulcerations may result, especially if applied to mucosal surfaces. Reversible alopecia has been reported with application to the beard area.[3] Most symptoms are self-healing, although postinflammatory hyperpigmentation may persist.[3]

No systemic adverse reactions have been reported after topical application of cidofovir. Only one report of a systemic effect after intralesional injection has been documented. After treating recurrent laryngeal papillomatosis with 2.5 mg/ml intralesional cidofovir, Snoeck et al[11] had one patient withdraw from the study because of 'precardial' complaints, although no cardiac abnormalities were noted. Long-term studies documenting the safety of topical and intralesional cidofovir are needed.

Table 16.1 Patient education sheet

What is cidofovir?
Cidofovir is a relatively new antiviral compound currently approved to treat cytomegalovirus retinitis in HIV patients. Recently, it has been shown to kill cells infected with human papillomavirus, the virus that causes warts.

What are the side effects?
Local reactions are common when using topical cidofovir. Burning, pain, redness, inflammation, and itching are frequently reported. Erosions and ulcerations can occur. Most symptoms are self-healing with little or no scarring.

How to use your cidofovir cream/gel
1. Clean affected area with soap and water; remove any excess dead skin from around the wart
2. Using a cotton-tipped applicator, carefully apply the cream/gel to the wart, avoiding the surrounding area of normal skin
3. Repeat this process twice a day or as your physician instructed
4. Call your physician if you have any problems such as excessive pain or ulceration

FAVORED TREATMENT METHODOLOGY

Informed consent should be obtained before initiating treatment of cidofovir. Side effects should be explained including local irritation and possible ulceration. As the topical formulation is not commercially available, cidofovir must be compounded in a base (Beeler or Dermavan base).[5] Patients should be instructed to apply 1% cidofovir cream/gel twice daily to cutaneous lesions or once a day for mucosal lesions. The cream should be applied with a cotton swab or wearing rubber gloves in a thin layer to cover the wart.[1] Follow-up should be scheduled for 1 or 2 weeks. No oral formulation is currently available.[9,14]

COURSE AND PROGNOSIS

Topical cidofovir commonly causes local irritation and inflammation. Erosions and ulcerations may occur. Regression of the lesion may be seen as early as a few days after initiation of treatment. Further studies are needed to determine success rates and optimal length of therapy.

CASE REPORTS

Case 1

Zabawski et al[4] reported a case of a 13-year-old girl who presented with a 3-year history of warts on her fingers. After unsuccessful attempts with several different therapies, including liquid nitrogen, cryosurgery, carbon dioxide laser ablation, and topical salicylic acid, the patient began daily 3% topical cidofovir in a Dermavan base. After only 2 weeks there was significant clinical improvement and after 10 weeks all warts had completely resolved. Adverse effects included 'slight irritation, and

minimal crusting' of the areas treated. The patient has since remained wart-free for 8 months.

Case 2

A 19-year-old college freshman had a 4-year history of warts on his left hand and elbow. He had attempted topical salicylic acid, cryotherapy, and cauterization in the past, with only temporary improvement of the lesions. On physical examination, the patient had two 2-mm verrucous lesions on his left middle finger and one 4.6-mm verrucous lesion on his left elbow. The patient was informed of the risks and benefits of treatment and consented. He was treated with 1% topical cidofovir to be applied twice daily. Within 1 week all three warts had clinically regressed to 50% of pretreatment size. The affected areas were scaly and irritated, and the patient complained of mild itching. After 7 more days of treatment, the warts had completely resolved with only minimal erythema remaining. No signs of recurrence were seen at a 9-month follow-up.

Case 3

A 40-year-old surgeon presented with a 2-year history of a 40-mm wart on the sole of his foot (Figure 16.3). He complained of pain and interference with daily function caused by the wart. Prior treatments included over-the-counter medications, cryotherapy with liquid nitrogen, and surgical excision on three occasions. After initial treatment, options were discussed and informed consent was obtained, the wart was circled, and he was injected intralesionally with cidofovir (Figure 16.4). The wart and surrounding skin became necrotic, requiring débridement on two occasions (Figure 16.5). The skin had returned completely to normal and the wart remained clear for 1 year after treatment (Figure 16.6).

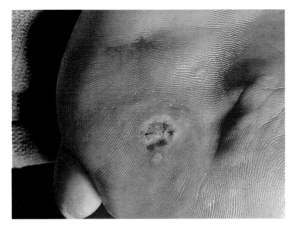

Figure 16.3
Wart on the foot of a surgeon, which recurred after three surgical excisions.

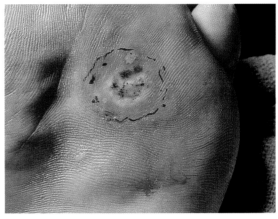

Figure 16.4
Wart on the foot that recurred after three surgical excisions now circled before injection with cidofovir.

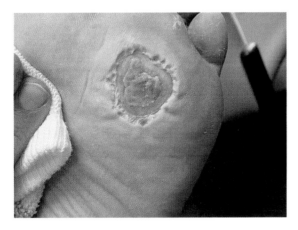

Figure 16.5
Site of treatment with cidofovir and paring. This picture was taken 3 weeks after initial injection with cidofovir.

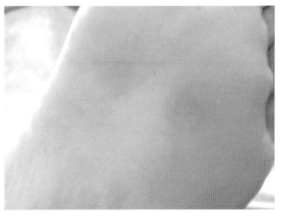

Figure 16.6
Same patient 1 year after one treatment with cidofovir.

REFERENCES

1. Snoeck R, Van Ranst M, Andrei G et al. Treatment of anogenital papillomavirus infections with an acyclic nucleoside phosphonate analogue. *N Engl J Med* 1995; **333**: 943–4.

2. Van Cutsem E, Snoeck R, Van Ranst M et al. Successful treatment of a squamous papilloma of the hypopharynx-esophagus by local injections of (1-[(*S*)-3-hydroxy-2-(phosphono-methoxy)-propyl]cytosine. *J Med Virol* 1995; **45**: 230–5.

3. Calista D. Topical cidofovir for severe cutaneous human papillomavirus and molluscum contagiosum infections in patients with HIV/AIDS. A pilot study. *J Eur Acad Dermatol Venereol* 2000; **14**: 484–8.

4. Zabawski EJ, Sands B, Goetz D, Naylor M, Cockerell CJ. Treatment of verruca vulgaris with topical cidofovir. *JAMA* 1997; **278**: 1236.

5. Zabawski EJ, Cockerell CJ. Topical and intralesional cidofovir: A review of pharmacology and therapeutic effects. *J Am Acad Dermatol* 1998; **39**: 741–5.

6. Gilman AG, Hardman JG, Limbird LE. In: *Goodman and Gilman's The Pharmacological Basis of Therapeutics*, 10th edn. McGraw-Hill Co., Inc., New York: 2001: 1429–30.

7. Johnson JA, Gangemi JD. Selective inhibition of human papillomavirus-induced cell proliferation by (1-[(S)-3-hydroxy-2-(phosphonomethoxy)-propyl]cytosine. *Antimicrob Agents Chemother* 1999; **43**: 1198–205.

8. Snoeck R, Wellens W, Desloovere C et al. Treatment of severe laryngeal papillomatosis with intralesional injections of cidofovir (1-[(S)-3-hydroxy-2-(phosphonomethoxy)-propyl]cytosine. *J Med Virol* 1998; **54**: 219–25.

9. Koonsaeng S, Verschraegen C, Freedman R et al. Successful treatment of recurrent vulvar intraepithelial neoplasia resistant to interferon and isotretinoin with cidofovir. *J Med Virol* 2001; **64**: 195–8.

10. Matteelli A, Beltrame A, Graifemberghi S et al. Efficacy and tolerability of topical 1% cidofovir cream for the treatment of external anogenital warts in HIV-infected persons. *Sex Transm Dis* 2001; **28**: 343–6.

11. Snoeck R, Bossens M, Parent D et al. Phase II double-blind, placebo-controlled study of the safety and efficacy of cidofovir topical gel for the treatment of patients with human papillomavirus infection. *Clin Infect Dis* 2001; **33**: 597–602.

12. Davis MD, Gostout BS, McGovern RM, Persing DH, Schut RL, Pittelkow MR. Large plantar wart caused by human papillomavirus-66 and resolution by topical cidofovir therapy. *J Am Acad Dermatol* 2000; **43**(2 Pt 2): 340–3.

13. Cook DJ, Guyatt GH, Lamparis A, Sackett DL, Goldberg RJ. Clinical recommendations using levels of evidence for antithrombotic agents. *Chest* 1995; **108**(suppl 4): 227S–30S.

14. Zabawski EJ. A review of topical and intralesional cidofovir. *Dermatol Online J* 2000; **6**: 3.

17 Intralesional immunotherapy

Sandra Marchese Johnson

Historical aspects • Basic science • Clinical studies • Adverse events • Favored treatment methodology • Course and prognosis • Case reports • References

Intradermal skin test antigens are readily available, having been commonly used for decades to establish the presence of intact cell-mediated immunity. Mumps and candida skin test antigens are most commonly used. They serve as positive control tests when used together with purified protein derivative (PPD) skin testing for tuberculosis.

HISTORICAL ASPECTS

Delayed type (type IV) hypersensitivity (DTH) is an immunological reaction that is primarily responsible for eradicating viral and fungal pathogens. DTH testing dates back to Edward Jenner in 1798. He noted that individuals re-vaccinated for cowpox developed an erythematous papule at the site of injection 24–72 hours after injection.[1] This was not appreciated in non-sensitized individuals before vaccination. Since then, DTH skin testing has become a routine measure of immunity to *Mycobacterium tuberculosis*. Induration is noted clinically when there is a 'positive reaction' to a skin test antigen. A negative test suggests that the patient has not been exposed, provided the patient is not anergic. Conversion from a negative to a positive test suggests recent infection with tuberculosis.

Control antigens are placed at the same time as a PPD. Humans are commonly exposed to the antigens chosen as controls. They are placed to test the proficiency and robustness of the cellular immune system. Therefore, there is a high likelihood of reactivity to these antigens, resulting in a meaningful and generally reliable comparison for the PPD antigen response. If both PPD and control tests are negative, the patient may be anergic and in this case a negative PPD test is less predictive of an absence of tuberculosis infection.[1–3]

Anergy may occur when a person has a limited number of functioning T cells or from another cause of immunodeficiency. There have been many studies to determine which antigens serve as the best controls. In 1113 patients who had skin tests placed on admission to a Texas hospital, 64% reacted to Candida and 52% to mumps.[4] Anergy has also been found to be a negative prognostic indicator in people with small-cell lung cancer. [5] Cimetidine, an H_2-receptor antagonist, discussed previously in Chapter 8, has been shown to increase response to skin test antigens. Cimetidine has also restored sensitivity to skin test antigens in people who have developed tolerance to the antigens. [6]

The United States Food and Drug Administration (FDA) has approved the use of mumps and Candida for anergy testing. They are used together but injected separately. Induration extending 5 mm from the intralesional injection site after 48–72 hours is considered a positive test. Mumps skin test antigen has been available for many years. The use of candida skin test antigen for anergy testing is relatively recent compared with mumps. Many pharmaceutical companies produce this antigen in a variety of concentrations and dilutions, and with various preservatives. As a result of the variations in preparations of candida skin test antigens, one should be cautious when interpreting skin test reactions to Candida.[3] The optimal concentration of candida antigen is unclear at this time.

BASIC SCIENCE

DTH responses are brisk immunological reactions to foreign antigens. They are T-cell mediated with specific targeting to the antigen. A secondary non-specific inflammation of both T cells and macrophages also occurs.

Mackaness[7] described the link between the induction of activated macrophage effector cells and DTH responses. While performing research with Listeria monocytogenes, he found that augmented macrophage antimicrobial activity was non-specific. Macrophages that are upregulated in response to infection by one bacterium also displayed increased activity against unrelated bacteria.[7] This is the rationale for injection of an antigen (mumps or Candida) that is likely to stimulate a DTH response within infected wart tissue.

There has been very limited research concerning the use of skin test antigens for the treatment of warts. However, we do possess a tremendous amount of experience and knowledge about the immunological mechanisms of DTH reactions induced by skin test antigens, tuberculosis and leprosy. In fact, the human body is thought to react to human papillomavirus (HPV) infection in a fashion that

is similar to the reaction to *Mycobacterium tuberculosis*. The natural history of tuberculosis and its various clinical manifestations are intimately related to the hosts' defenses. A brisk host response helps to control or abolish infections with mycobacteria and HPV. As neither mycobacteria nor HPV is capable of producing classic endo- or exotoxins, many of the clinical manifestations (or lack thereof) are mediated by the host during the 'immune' response to the infection, rather than being the direct effects of the infectious organisms. [1–3,7]

The pathophysiological basis of DTH reactions in sensitized individuals with normal immune status can be summarized as follows: a known antigen is placed intradermally using the Mantoux method. A cascade of events occurs at the site of antigen injection, commencing with mononuclear cells accumulating at the postcapillary venules 4 hours after injection. Macrophages engulf the antigen and release lymphokines that attract T lymphocytes. The macrophages then process phagocytosed antigens to these lymphocytes, initiating an expansion of clones that recognize various epitopes as well as additional non-specific recruitment of T cells and leukocytes. These lymphocytes elaborate further cytokines which activate macrophages, enhancing their function. These macrophages are free to attack viral and fungal organisms in the area. Permeability of vessels is increased, leading to edema and fibrin deposition. Furthermore T cells and macrophage accumulation, together with edema, produce the clinically recognized induration 24–48 hours after injection. In the case of tuberculosis, skin test reactivity develops 4–6 weeks after infection, although intervals of up to 20 weeks can occur.[8] This may explain the time period required to induce the rejection of warts in patients treated intralesionally with skin test antigens.

Contact sensitivity is a type of DTH in which the antigen is applied topically to the epidermis, with subsequent uptake by Langerhans' cells. An example of contact sensitivity is exposure to urushiol from the poison ivy plant. In this theory, an antigen will not elicit contact sensitivity when Langerhans' cell function is diminished or total number of Langerhans' cells are reduced as a result of localized or systemic immunosuppression caused by corticosteroids, cytoreductive chemotherapy or ultraviolet light exposure. The relative importance of Langerhans' cells in type IV hypersensitivity induced by intradermal injection of antigen is unknown, although Langerhans' cells can be identified among spindle cells of the dermis.[2]

One potential difficulty in using intralesional immunotherapy lies in the fact that DTH reactions may be decreased in people with warts, e.g. tuberculin sensitivity in BCG-immunized children with common warts was found to be reduced when compared with children without warts.[9]

CLINICAL STUDIES

There has been only one prospective clinical trial published in the English literature using intralesional skin test antigens.[10] One retrospective chart review has been published.[11] Lectures about the treatment of warts with skin test antigens have also been presented at scientific meetings.[12] In the prospective clinical trial, intralesional skin test antigens were injected into one wart. Clearing of the treated wart was demonstrated in 74% of participants, as opposed to clearing of 55% of warts treated with cryotherapy. In both groups, one treatment was administered every 3 weeks; 78% of the participants with clearing of the target wart with intralesional skin test antigens also experienced clearing of untreated anatomically distant warts. Regression of distant warts has not been demonstrated with any other therapy. The significance of distant wart regression is not yet known.[10] It does, however, imply acquisition of HPV-directed immunity.

In the retrospective study, 70% of patients treated with intralesional injection of candida skin test antigen experienced clearance of their warts within 8 weeks of treatment. These authors also noted that 86% of people treated were satisfied with the treatment and 82% would repeat the treatment if needed.[11]

We give the treatment of intralesional immunotherapy a level of evidence rating of II because of one randomized clinical trial.

ADVERSE EVENTS

In contrast to DTH skin testing, Candida and mumps skin test antigens often do not cause a visible reaction at the site of the wart even in patients who showed prior positive skin test reactions. In fact, in my personal experience of treating more than 500 individuals with this modality, 3% have demonstrated erythema or induration in the wart (unpublished results). One explanation may be that the thickened epidermis of the wart disguise any underlying inflammatory reaction. Approximately 3% of individuals will experience flu-like symptoms consisting of fevers, chills and myalgias that start 4 hours after treatment and last no more than 24 hours (unpublished data).

FAVORED TREATMENT METHODOLOGY

1. Physical examination to determine that the lesion to be treated is, in fact, a wart; a biopsy is recommended if in doubt
2. Place intradermal skin test by intradermal injection of mumps (Aventis Pasteur, Swiftwater, PA) and Candida (Hollister-Stier, Spokane, WA) test antigen preparations 0.1 ml in the left and right forearms respectively (Figures 17.1–17.4).

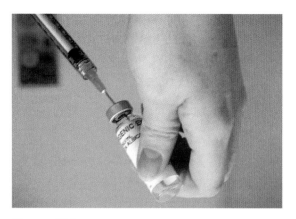

Figure 17.1
Physician drawing up 0.1 ml of candida skin
test antigen into a syringe.

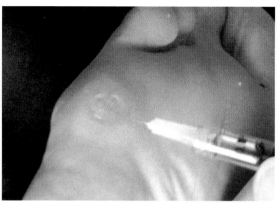

Figure 17.2
Physician injecting one portion of a plantar wart.

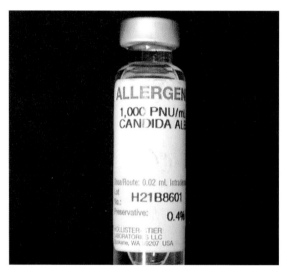

Figure 17.3
A vial of candida skin test antigen manufactured
by Hollister-Steir in Spokane, WA.

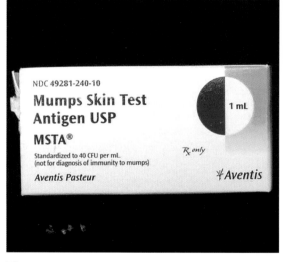

Figure 17.4
A box containing a vial of mumps skin test
antigen manufactired by Aventis Pasteur in
Swiftwater, PA.

3. Determine skin test reaction; the presence
    or absence and size of the ensuing reactions
    are noted after 48–72 hours. Determination
    of a positive reaction necessitates erythema
    and induration of at least 5 mm in diameter.
    If no reaction occurs, intralesional treatment
    of warts is not initiated. If a positive reaction
    occurs, proceed to step 4

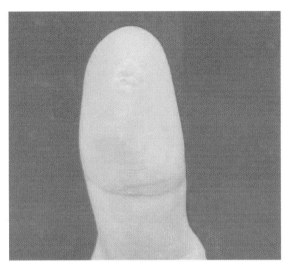

Figure 17.5
A verrucous papule is noted on the thumb.

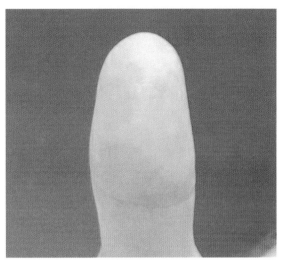

Figure 17.6
The same thumb as seen in Figure 17.5 after therapy with intralesional skin test antigens.

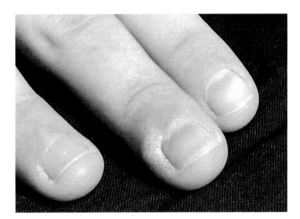

Figure 17.7
Verrucous papule on right middle and index fingers, involving the lateral nail fold.

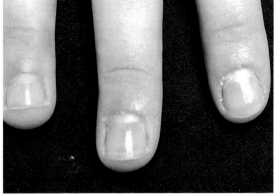

Figure 17.8
Resolved periungual wart shown in Figure 17.7 after two treatments with intralesional candida skin test antigen.

4. Administer first treatment with intralesional, not intradermal, injection of mumps or candida antiserum into the largest wart in a volume determined by the size of the test reaction; 0.3 ml injected with test site induration of 5–20 mm, 0.2 ml injected with test site induration of 20–40 mm, and 0.1 ml with test site induration of

> 40 mm. This approach is used to decrease the incidence of flu-like reactions (Figures 17.5–17.8)

5. Re-evaluate and re-treat if needed every 3 weeks as long as the wart persists. If there is no clinical response after three or four treatments, an alternative therapeutic modality is recommended

A patient information sheet can be helpful (Table 17.1).

COURSE AND PROGNOSIS

Initial reports note a decreased incidence of recurrence after treatment with intralesional skin test antigens compared with other therapies. It is theorized that this treatment stimulates long-term immunity against HPV. This therapy is a new addition to the armamentarium against warts and long-term data are not available.

CASE REPORTS

Case 1

A 19-year-old healthy white man presented with multiple warts. His warts had been present for 3 years. Prior unsuccessful treatments included over-the-counter salicylic acid, cryotherapy, surgical excision and topical imiquimod. He had an unremarkable past and family medical history. On physical examination a 1-cm verrucous plaque was present on his right index finger. Multiple smaller warts were also present on his left leg, left arm and left little finger (Figure 17.9). A diagnosis of verruca vulgaris was made. After discussing treatment options, the patient elected to be treated with intralesional skin test antigen immunotherapy. Mumps and candida skin test antigens were placed intradermally using the Mantoux method, which is similar to the placement of a PPD skin test. After 72 hours there was no induration at the site of the mumps

Table 17.1 Patient education

Intralesional immunotherapy for the treatment of warts

Mumps skin test antigen and candida skin test antigen are FDA (Food and Drug Administration) approved for intradermal (into the skin) injection to determine whether your body can react to them and recognize them as foreign. This is also referred to as anergy testing. Once it is known that your body can recognize the antigen as abnormal, it can be injected into a wart to stimulate your body to recognize abnormal features of the wart. It is hoped that your own immunity will attack and clear the wart. This is a relatively new approach and is not an FDA-approved treatment for warts.

This treatment will be repeated approximately every 3 weeks until your wart is gone or until you decide to stop this treatment. Usually about three to five treatments are needed to notice a reduction in your warts.

There are several benefits of this treatment. Only one wart needs to be treated and all of the warts may disappear. The treatment is relatively painless.

The side effects of this treatment include itching, redness or swelling at the site of the injection. Less than 5% of people develop flu-like symptoms (fever, chills, muscle aches), which last about 24 hours after the injection, or develop itching, swelling or redness at the site of injection. Also, unfortunately, not everyone who is treated with skin test antigens will notice their warts disappear.

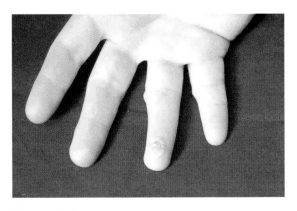

Figure 17.9
A large verrucous papule is noted on the right ring finger.

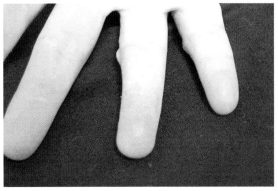

Figure 17.10
Resolution of the wart in Figure 17.9 is noted after injection with intralesional skin test antigen.

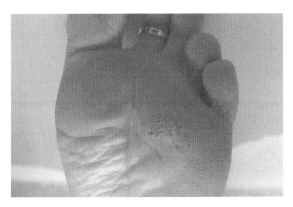

Figure 17.11
A large cluster of exophytic and endophytic verrucous papules consistent with plantar warts are noted on the sole of the foot.

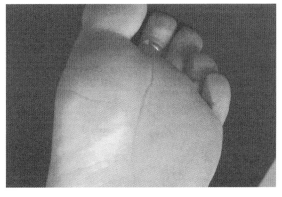

Figure 17.12
Resolution of all wart pictured in Figure 17.11 is noted without residual scar after treatment with intralesional immunotherapy.

skin test antigen injection and a 5-mm induration at the site of the candida skin test antigen injection. Then 0.3 ml of candida skin test antigen was injected into the wart on the index finger on the right hand. He returned every 3 weeks for re-evaluation and re-treatment. When he returned for the third injection, the treated wart and all distant warts had resolved. Normal skin markings returned and there was no scarring. The patient returned to this clinic 2 years later for treatment of acne and commented that all his warts were still resolved (Figure 17.10). No new warts had developed.

Case 2

A 24-year-old woman presented complaining of warts for 2 years. Prior therapy consisted of cryotherapy with liquid nitrogen and topical salicylic acid. Her past medical history was unremarkable. On physical examination she was a healthy-appearing white woman. She had a 12 × 20 mm verrucous plaque and a 5 × 5 mm papule on her right sole (Figure 17.11). There was also a group of six 5-mm verrucous papules on her left sole and a 3 mm papule on her left heel. A clinical diagnosis of plantar warts was made. Treatment options were discussed with the patient. The patient elected to be treated with immunotherapy with intralesional skin test antigens. Mumps and candida skin test antigens were placed using the Mantoux method; 72 hours later she returned with 17-mm induration at the site of the candida skin test placement and minimal erythema at the site of the mumps skin test placement. A 5-mm verruca was injected with 0.2 ml of candida skin test antigen. She returned for re-evaluation and treatment every 3 weeks. When she returned for her third treatment all the warts had disappeared (Figure 17.12). There was no scarring.

REFERENCES

1. Meltzer MS, Nacy CA. Delayed-type hypersensitivity and the induction of activated, cytotoxic macrophages. In: Paul WE (ed.), *Fundamental Immunology*. New York: Raven Press, 1989: 765–8.

2. Abbas AK, Lichtman AH, Pober JS. *Cellular and Molecular Immunology*. Philadelphia: WB Saunders Co., 1991: 245–50.

3. Centers for Disease Control and Prevention. Anergy skin testing and preventative therapy for HIV-infected persons: revised recommendations. *MMWR* 1997; **46**: RR-15.

4. Wright PW, Crutcher JE, Holiday DB. Selection of skin test antigens to evaluate PPD anergy. *J Fam Pract* 1995; **41**: 59–64.

5. Johnston-Early A, Cohen MH, Fossieck BE Jr et al. Delayed hypersensitivity skin testing as a prognostic indicator in patients with small cell lung cancer. *Cancer* 1983; **52**: 1395–400.

6. Kumar A. Cimetidine: an immunomodulator. *Drug Intell Clin Pharm* 1990; **24**: 289–95.

7. Mackaness GB. Delayed hypersensitivity and the mechanism of cellular resistance to infection. In: Amos B (ed.), *Progress in Immunology*. New York: Academic Press, 1971: 413.

8. Iseman MD. Tuberculosis. In: Bennet JC, Plum F (eds), *Cecil Textbook of Internal Medicine*, 20th edn. Philadelphia: WB Saunders Co., 1996: 1683.

9. Brodersen I, Genner J, Brodthagen H. Tuberculin sensitivity in BCG-vaccinated children with common warts. *Acta Dermato-Venereol* 1974; **54**: 291–2.

10. Johnson SM, Roberson PK, Horn TD. Intralesional injection of mumps or candida antigens: a novel immnotherapy for warts. *Arch Dermatol* 2001; **137**: 451–5.

11. Phillips RC, Ruhl TS, Pfenninger JL, Garber MR. Treatment of warts with candida antigen injection. *Arch Dermatol* 2000; **136**: 1274–5.

12. Brunk D. Injection of Candida antigen works on warts. *Skin and Allergy News* 1999; **30**: 5.

18 Other office-based therapies: photodynamic therapy and hypnosis

Huwaida E Mansour and Robert T Brodell

Photodynamic therapy • Historical aspects • Basic science • Clinical evidence • Favored treatment methodology • Adverse effects • Case report • Hypnosis • Historical aspects • Basic science • Clinical evidence • Favored treatment methodology • Adverse effects • Case report • References

In addition to the wart therapies based in the doctor's surgery that have been reviewed in previous chapters, two other procedures have been used widely enough to warrant discussion – photodynamic therapy and hypnosis.

PHOTODYNAMIC THERAPY

Since its discovery in the early 1900s, photodynamic therapy (PDT) has been used in the treatment of pre-malignant and malignant skin conditions such as superficial squamous cell carcinoma, basal cell carcinoma, and actinic keratosis with varying degrees of success. More recently, investigational studies have proposed that PDT be used for non-oncological conditions such as psoriasis and HPV-related dermatoses. PDT aims to destroy pathologically altered cells through an interaction between absorbed light and either a systemic or topically applied photosensitizing agent. 5-Aminolevulinic acid (ALA), an 'endogenous' topical sensitizer, has been the most widely studied photosensitizing agent. PDT with topical ALA application, followed by irradi-ation using non-laser light, is a novel approach to treating recalcitrant warts when traditional therapies fail.

HISTORICAL ASPECTS

In 1904, Von Tappeiner discovered photodynamic therapy, using photosensitization followed by irradiation with visible light, to cause tissue destruction.[1] The following year Von Tappeiner and Jesionek discovered that human skin malignancies improved after the application of a 5% solution of eosin dye and subsequent exposure to lamps or sunlight.[2] Auler and Banzer, in 1947, were the first to use systemic PDT with intravenous hemato-porphyrin derivatives (HpD) of human and animal tumors as photosensitizers.[3] In 1978, Dougherty et al[4] performed the first study using intravenous HpD on human malignancies. Systemic HpD was, however, found to have significant unwanted side effects, most particularly prolonged cutaneous photosensitivity.[5] Consequently, research efforts were expanded to test different photosensitizing agents that could be applied topically. Kennedy et al,[6] in 1990, were the first to publish a study that yielded positive results in the treatment of basal cell carcinoma using topical ALA-PDT. Psoriasis has also been sucessfully treated using PDT.[7,8]

BASIC SCIENCE

The utility of PDT in the treatment of warts is rooted in the destructive effects of light that is focused on a specific cell type, while avoiding damage to surrounding structures. The photo-dynamic reaction excites photosensitizers (mainly porphyrins) with visible light in the presence of oxygen, yielding free radicals.[9] Cytotoxic species induce targeted cellular destruction.[9] This effect is produced by using sensitizing molecules via intravenous adminis-tration, or direct topical or intralesional applica-tion; these molecules selectively enter targeted cells. Most sensitizing molecules are not endogenous to the human body. HpD has been the focus of most of the published work but, as a result of its lack of selectivity for skin tumors and long-lasting photosensitivity, its utility has proved limited. In contrast, topical administration of 'endogenous' sensitizers such as ALA induce the synthesis of photo-sensitizers (protoporphyrin IX) in target tissues.[10]

5-Aminolevulinic acid has several properties that render it suited to PDT. Penetration of the skin is enhanced because it is a small hydrophilic molecule. When given intra-venously, ALA results in the accumulation of protoporphyrin IX in epithelial and mucosal tissues, but not in muscle, connective tissue, or cartilage.[11] In addition, porphyrins are made in much higher concentrations in epidermal cells, compared with fibroblasts, myocytes, or endothelial cells.[10] ALA is a precursor in the metabolic pathway of heme synthesis that produces protoporphyrin IX.[11] Protoporphyrin

IX accumulates in cells and produces a pink–red fluorescence when activated by either blue or violet light.[11] Pre-malignant and malignant tumors may interfere with heme metabolism and result in ALA-induced proto-porphyrin IX being accumulated in greater amounts than in normal tissue.[11] The mecha-nisms explaining the effectiveness of PDT on other dermatological conditions are under investigation.

CLINICAL EVIDENCE

Stender et al[12] treated 250 recalcitrant hand and foot warts in 30 patients using 20% ALA, in an oil-in-water emulsion applied topically under occlusion for 5 hours. The warts were irradiated using either a red, white, or blue light once or three times within 10 days.[12] Recalcitrant warts were defined as those that were long standing (average 3 years) and resisted treatment with a variety of modalities such as cryotherapy, caustic agents, superficial X-rays, excision, curettage, and laser treat-ments.[12] More than 70% of warts regressed in the group treated with white light using three treatments.[12] At the 1-year follow-up, none of the patients had any recurrent warts. In 2000, Stender et al[13] published a randomized, double-masked study of 232 foot and hand warts in 45 patients. Warts treated with PDT had 20% ALA in a cream base applied topically to pared-down warts using occlusive dressings, followed 4 hours later with broadband (590–700 nm) red light (Waldmann PDT 1200) delivered at 50 mW/cm^2 to a total fluence of 70 J/cm^2. Warts assigned to the 'placebo-PDT' (vehicle + light) received the identical vehicle without ALA, under occlusive dressing for 4 hours, followed by identical broadband red light illumination.[13] Treatments were repeated after 1 and 2 weeks.[13] Warts persisting at week 7 received three more ALA-PDT or vehicle + light treatments, again at weekly intervals.[13] Follow-up at 1 month revealed a 98% reduction in the wart area for the ALA-PDT-treated group.[13] The placebo group showed only a 52% regression in the wart area.[13] At the 2-month follow-up, a 100% reduction in the wart area was successfully achieved in the treatment group.

These studies with topical ALA-PDT appear to be promising. Further double-masked, randomized controlled trials will be required to confirm the effectiveness of PDT in patients with recalcitrant foot and hand warts, and to elucidate the most effective photosensitizing agents, concentration, vehicle, phototherapy source, and dosimetry. Using our Modified Evidence-based Medicine System (see Chapter 19), we rate the evidence for ALA-PDT as level I. It remains to be seen if this somewhat new and expensive technology will be widely accepted for the treatment of warts.

FAVORED TREATMENT METHODOLOGY

This treatment is in the early stages of investigation and no specific method is recommended at this time.

ADVERSE EFFECTS

As noted earlier, systemic PDT can result in prolonged cutaneous photosensitivity after only a single treatment. The first literature reference to cutaneous photosensitization resulting from administration of exogenous ALA appears to be the observation made by Berlin et al.[14] They reported that oral administration of ALA to humans was rapidly followed by a transient tingling or burning sensation and erythema of light-exposed skin.[14] To minimize generalized cutaneous photosensitivity, topical applications of sensitizers such as ALA for localized diseases such as warts seems prudent. The only significant acute side effect of topical ALA-PDT described by patients is a 'stinging', 'tingling', or 'burning' pain during and shortly after irradiation. Local skin reactions reported also included edema, erythema, and/or discoloration. The long-term effects are still being studied but could include all known effects of phototoxic damage such as the induction of skin tumors, although it is anticipated that the focused effects of PDT minimize the chance of these effects.

CASE REPORT

A 28-year-old white man presented with a 2-year history of a wart on the plantar surface of the right fourth toe. Transient improvement was noted after liquid nitrogen cryotherapy (30-second freeze time) on four occasions, cantharidin–salicylic acid–podophyllum under occlusion for 2 hours on four occasions, and vascular lesion laser therapy on five occasions with treatment every 3–4 weeks over a 1-year period. Transient improvement was, however, followed by enlargement and the wart was 8 × 9 mm in diameter when first examined at our surgery (Figure 18.1a). Treatment was started with topical ALA-PDT using a red light (Waldmann PDT 1200 L) delivered at 100 mW/cm^2 to a total fluence of 075.0 J/cm^2 (one treatment every 2 weeks for four treatments). Salicylic acid 12% in collodion base was applied each morning at home and the wart was filed with an emery board each evening. After 2 weeks the wart appeared unchanged except for the white discoloration of the wart caused by the salicylic acid treatment (Figure 18.1b). One week after the fourth PDT treatment, the wart was 70% improved (Figure 18.1c). Six weeks after

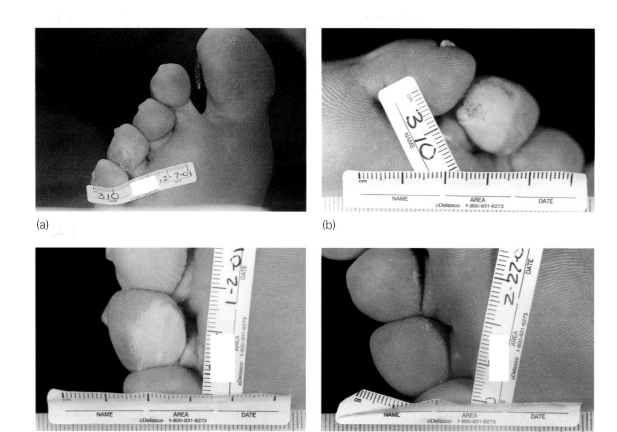

(a)

(b)

(c)

(d)

Figure 18.1

(a) A wart of 8 × 9 mm diameter persists on the plantar aspect of the right fourth toe despite previous treatment with liquid nitrogen cryotherapy, cantharidin–salicylic acid–podophyllum treatments, and vascular lesion laser therapy. (b) Two weeks after an initial treatment with photodynamic therapy (PDT), the wart is essentially unchanged. The white color is caused by daily adjunctive salicylic acid home treatments. (c) One week after the fourth PDT treatment, the wart appears to have disappeared. There was no further treatment with either PDT or salicylic acid. (d) Six weeks after the fourth PDT treatment, the skin on the right fourth toe appears entirely normal.

treatment ended the wart was clear (Figure 18.1d).

utilized but hypnosis has been studied most extensively. This approach to the treatment of warts is based on of the power of suggestion.

HYPNOSIS

Non-pharmacologic treatments of warts have been studied widely. Many methods have been

HISTORICAL ASPECTS

Various studies published over the past 70 years have described the success of hypnosis and the power of suggestion in the treatment of verruca vulgaris and verruca plana. Research investigating hypnosis as a potential treatment modality for warts can be traced back to as early as the 1930s. Contributions have been made by many authors, including McDowell, and Obermayer and Greenson in the 1940s, Asher and Allington in the 1950s, Ullman and Dudek in the 1960s, and Surnam et al in the 1970s.[15–20.] Sinclair-Geiben and Chalmers,[21] in 1959, conducted a landmark study in which they recruited 14 patients with bilateral common warts and exposed them to hypnotic induction consisting of repeated suggestions of relaxation, drowsiness, and sleep. After five treatments within a 3-month period, 9 of 10 hypnotized patients reported improvement of the warts on the treated side, as opposed to no clinical regression of the warts on the untreated side.[21] These studies laid the foundation for more recent placebo-controlled observational studies.

BASIC SCIENCE

The exact mechanism by which hypnosis and suggestion cause wart regression has not been elucidated. Hypnosis and the power of suggestion are thought to affect the host–virus relationship via psychological factors that lead to a systemic physiological alteration in the microenvironment of virally infected cells. Other investigators such as Ullman believe that the power of suggestion causes autonomic changes which result in wart resolution.[19] A definitive scientific explanation of the effects of hypnosis that can lead to selective regression on only one side of the body requires further investigation.

CLINICAL EVIDENCE

Surman et al[20] performed a noteworthy study in 1973. They hypnotized 17 patients with bilateral common or flat warts weekly for five sessions, and the suggestion was made that the warts would disappear on one side only. Within 3 months, 9 of the 17 hypnotized patients showed a regression of their warts on the treated side.[20] In addition, they examined an untreated control group consisting of seven patients and found that none of them had noticed any regression of their warts after 3 months.[20]

Spanos et al[22] conducted two experiments in 1988. In the first experiment, 63 patients with warts on one or both hands were randomly assigned to one of three groups: the hypnotic suggestion group, the 'cold laser' placebo group, or a 'no treatment' control group; 22 patients received hypnosis whereas 24 patients had cold laser treatments. Both groups had their warts counted and were asked to return in 6 weeks for follow-up. The 17 remaining individuals were informed that they were placed on a waiting list and should return in 6 weeks for treatment. At the end of the 6 weeks, all the participants had their warts counted again. One or more warts cleared in half of the patients treated with hypnotic suggestion, whereas only 6 of 24 from the 'cold laser' placebo group and 2 of 17 patients from the 'no treatment' control group reported wart resolution.[22] This small controlled experiment provides evidence that hypnotic suggestion was more effective than placebo or 'no treatment'.[22] In the second experiment, hypnotic and non-hypnotic participants given identical suggestions were equally likely to exhibit wart regression and more likely to show this effect than no treatment controls.[22] Moreover, in 1990, Spanos et al.[23] compared hypnosis against salicylic acid, placebo, and no treatment in a double-masked placebo controlled trial of 40 individuals.[23] Six weeks after the treatment period only the hypnotic participants had significantly fewer warts. The acid, placebo treatment, and no treatment group showed no significant change.[23]

Using our Modified Evidence-based Medicine System (see Chapter 19) we rate the evidence for hypnosis in the treatment of warts as a level II based on the clinical evidence presented above. Clearly, hypnosis for the treatment of warts needs greater scientific investigation. We find it difficult to recommend the widespread adoption of this therapy, which, above all others in this book, is rooted in the expertise of the individual practitioner.

FAVORED TREATMENT METHODOLOGY

The evidence does not favor a specific treatment modality. Hypnosis involves several to many sessions in the surgery with a qualified psychiatrist, psychologist, or other experienced physician and a willing participant who has the necessary traits to be hypnotized. Therapists utilize a variety of procedures to induce the hypnotic state and enhance the effectiveness of suggestion.

ADVERSE EFFECTS

Once a patient becomes hypnotized he or she is dependent on the therapist, so a positive or negative transference may develop. The therapist must respect the patient and focus on the goal of the hypnotic session.

CASE REPORT

Currently, we have no experience with hypnosis in our surgery. Case reports demonstrating the utility of hypnosis are available in several published articles.[19,24]

REFERENCES

1. Von Tappeiner H, Jodlbauer A. Uber die Wirkungen der photodynamischen (fluore-scierend) Stoffe auf Protozoen and Enzyme. *Arch Klin Med* 1904; **80**: 427–87.

2. Jesionek A, von Tappeiner H. Zur Behandlung der Hautcarcinome mit fluore-scierenden Stoffen. *Dtsch Arch Klin Med* 1905; **85**: 223–7.

3. Auler H, Banzer G. Untersuchungen über die Rolle der Porphyrine bie geschwulstkranken Meschen und Tieren. *A Krebforsch* 1942; **53**: 65–8.

4. Dougherty TJ, Kaufman JE, Goldfarb A et al. Photoradiation therapy for the treatment of malignant tumors. *Cancer Res* 1978; **38**: 2628–35.

5. Wooten RS, Smith KC, Ahlquist DA et al. Prospective study of cutaneous phototoxicity after systemic hematoporphyrin derivative. *Lasers Surg Med* 1988; **8**: 294–300.

6. Kennedy JC, Pottier RH, Pross DC et al. Photodynamic therapy with endogenous protoporhyrin IX: Basic principles and present clinical experience. *J Photochem Photobiol B: Biol* 1990; **6**: 143–8.

7. Weinstein GD, McCullough JL, Jeffes EW. Photodynamic therapy (PDT0 of psoriasis with topical delta aminolevulinic acid (ALA): A pilot dose ranging study. *Photodermatol Photoimmunol Photomed* 1994; **10**: 92.

8. Boehncke WH, Sterry W, Kaufmann R. Treatment of psoriasis by topical photodynamic therapy with polychromatic light. *Lancet* 1994; **343**: 801–2.

9. Pass HI. Photodynamic therapy in oncology: Mechanisms and clinical use. *J Natl Cancer Inst* 1993; **85**: 443–56.

10. Kennedy JC, Pottier RH. Endogenous protoporphyrin IX , a clinically useful photosenitizer for photodynamic therapy. *J Photochem Photobiol B: Biol* 1992; **14**: 275–92.

11. Kennedy JC, Marcus SL, Pottier RH. Photodynamic therapy (PDT) and photodiagnosis (PD) using endogenous photosensitization induced by 5-aminolevulinic acid (ALA): Current clinical and developmental status. *J Clin Laser Med Surg* 1996; **14**: 59–66.

12. Stender IM, Lock-Anderson J, Wulf HC.

Recalcitrant hand and foot warts successfully treated with photodynamic therapy with topical 5-aminolaevulinic acid: a pilot study. *Clin Exp Dermatol* 1999; **24**: 154–9.

13. Stender IM, Ha R, Fogh H et al. Photodynamic therapy with 5-aminolaevulinic acid or placebo for recalcitrant foot and hand warts: randomized double-blind trial. *Lancet* 2000; **355**: 963–6.

14. Berlin NI, Neuberger A, Scott JJ. The metabolism of delta-aminolaevulinic acid. Normal pathways, studied with the aid of ^{14}C. *Biochem J* 1956; **64**: 90–100.

15. McDowell H. Juvenile warts removed with the use of hypnotic suggestions. *Bull Menninger Clin* 1949; **13**: 124–6.

16. Obermayer ME, Greenson RR. Treatment by suggestion of verrucae planae of the face. *Psychosom Med* 1949; **11**: 163–4.

17. Asher R. Respectable hypnosis. *BMJ* 1956; **1**: 309–13.

18. Allington HV. Review of psychotherapy of warts. *Arch Dermatol Syphilol* 1952; **66**: 316–26.

19. Ullman M, Dudek S. On the psyche and warts: II. Hypnotic suggestion and warts. *Psychosom Med* 1960; **22**: 68–76.

20. Surman OS, Gottlieb SK, Hackett TP, Silverberg EL. Hypnosis in the treatment of warts. *Arch Gen Psychiatry* 1973; **28**: 439–41.

21. Sinclair-Gieben AHC, Chalmers D. Evaluation of treatment of warts by hypnosis. *Lancet* 1959; **2**: 480–2.

22. Spanos NP, Stenstrom RJ, Johnston JC. Hypnosis, placebo, and suggestion in the treatment of warts. *Psychosom Med* 1988; **50**: 245–60.

23. Spanos NP, Williams V, Gwynn M. Effects of hypnotic, placebo and salicylic acid treatments on wart regression. *Psychosom Med* 1990; **52**: 109–11.

24. Johnson RF, Barber TX. Hypnosis, suggestions, and warts: an experimental investigation implicating the importance of 'believed efficacy'. *Am J Clin Hypn* 1978; **20**: 165–174.

19 Evidence-based medicine

Sandra Marchese Johnson

Prior attempts at EBM for warts • EBM for warts in 2002 • References

In 1951, Lemprière declared: 'Of all the futile disorders of the skin, it would be hard to find any that are regarded with greater contempt by the lay public and yet capable of resisting a greater variety of treatment than the group of papillary lesions commonly known as warts'.[1] Unfortunately, even in view of the superb research conducted in the last 50 years, which is reviewed in this book, this statement has not been disproved.

Treatment recommendations can be based on art, personal experience, personal preference, community standards of care, anecdotes or expert opinion. The best treatment recommendations are, however, based on a thorough review of the literature to produce an approach rooted in the best scientific evidence available. Of course, when different individuals analyse data, there may be conflicting recommendations. Use of a common rating system, and publication of recommendations and the evidence on which they are based, may resolve such conflicts.

Our goal in writing this book is not to provide a tutorial on evidence-based medicine (EBM) nor to dictate a treatment approach for the warts of individual patients. Our intent is rather to provide and analyze the most current information available for the treatment of human papillomavirus (HPV) infections. The condensed information focuses on clinical trials, especially randomized clinical trials. We have modified currently available tools for analyzing the strength of evidence upon which treatment decisions are based. Our system most closely resembles the Oxford Center for Evidence-based Medicine levels of evidence. We do not provide grades of recommendation preferring to allow the reader to make an informed decision about choice of therapy based primarily on the strength of evidence.[2–4] The lack of available evidence does not imply that a method of treatment should not be employed, nor does a high level of evidence rating necessarily mean that particular therapy is the best therapy for the individual patient which you are treating. Each treatment decision should be based on the experience of the physician, patient preference, and the application of evidence-based medicine. Table 19.1 provides the rationale for each level of reference. We aim for the data presented to entice the reader to review the literature presented and make their own judgement which we hope will validate ourt efforts. Of course, the debate will continue as new evidence leads to further adjustments in the level of evidence assigned to a specific treatment.

PRIOR ATTEMPTS AT EBM FOR WARTS

Efforts to develop an empirical approach to the treatment of warts are not new. The American Academy of Dermatology's Committee on

Table 19.1 Levels of evidence

Level of evidence	Description
I	RCTs with low false-positive (alpha) and low false-negative (beta) errors; high power; large trials with clear-cut results; all or none case series; or meta-analysis in which the lower limit of the CI for the treatment effect exceeds the minimal clinically important benefit
II	RCTs with high false-positive (alpha) and/or high false-negative (beta) errors; low power; single RCT in which the CI for the treatment overlaps the minimal clinically important benefit; or outcomes research
III	Non-randomized concurrent cohort comparisons between contemporaneous patients
IV	Non-randomized historical cohort comparisons
V	Case series without controls; small studies; anecdotal reports; or expert opinion

RCT: randomized clinical trial; CI: confidence interval.
Adapted from the literature.[2-4]

Table 19.2 Home therapies

Therapy	Level of evidence
Salicylic acid	I
Imiquimod for genital warts	I
Imiquimod for cutaneous non-genital warts	IV
Podophyllotoxin for genital warts	I
Cimetidine	V
Retinoids (oral and topical)	V
Heat therapy	IV
Supportive homeopathy	V

Guidelines of Care has established indications for the treatment of warts. These include: (1) desire of the patient for therapy, (2) symptoms of pain, bleeding, itching or burning, (3) disabling or disfiguring lesions, (4) large numbers or large size of lesions, (5) desire to prevent spread to unblemished skin of patient or others and (6) immunocompromised condi-tion.[5] We are in agreement with these recom-mendations.

The Cochrane Database of Systematic Reviews states that the first-line therapy of non-genital cutaneous warts is salicylic acid; the second-line treatment is cryotherapy; third-line therapies include immunotherapy, intra-lesional bleomycin injections, surgical excision, or curettage and cautery. In view of the complexities involved in the treatment of warts of different sizes, shapes and subtypes in different locations, this approach is too simplistic. We do agree, however, with the conclusion that a systematic review of all treatments is needed.[6] One of our aims with this book has been to attempt that review. Of course, in a world of evolving science, there is never as much scientific evidence to support day-to-day practice as we would like. It is hoped that future studies will include more head-to-head comparisons with careful design to determine both response rates and recurrence rates. Cost-effectiveness and potential scarring are two other aspects of wart therapy that should be evaluated.[6]

Sterling et al[7] provided a summary of treatments for warts published in 2001. They also applied evidence-based medicine to their review. They found good evidence to support the use of cryotherapy in the treatment of warts, and fair evidence to support the use of photodynamic therapy, salicylic acid, bleomycin and retinoids, but poor evidence to support the use of formaldehyde, thermocautery, glutaraldehyde, chemical cautery, CO_2 laser, pulsed dye laser and topical sensitization. In addition, they found fair evidence to reject the use of cimetidine and oral homoeopathy, and insufficient evidence to review podophyllin, folk remedies, hypnosis, heat treatments, interferon or imiquimod. They charged the dermatological community with several tasks, the most relevant of which is to find the best treatment regimen for warts using liquid nitrogen cryotherapy and topical salicylic acid.

A questionnaire sent to genitourinary physicians established the standard of care in England and Wales in 1992. Wardropper and Wooley[8] found the first-line treatment for anogenital warts to be podophyllin and the second-line treatment cryotherapy. An EBM review for the treatment of genital warts was published in 2001. The author concluded that

podophyllotoxin, imiquimod and intralesional interferon can clear warts better than placebo. Adequate randomized clinical trials were not found comparing placebo with cryotherapy, electrosurgery, surgical excision or laser surgery.[12]

EBM FOR WARTS IN 2003

Our review of the literature on the treatment of warts is not all inclusive. Although we provide information on basic science, we do not attempt to discuss vaccine therapies for warts. There is little evidence of an effective vaccine in the literature that has been

Table 19.3 Therapies administered in the physician's office

Therapy	Level of evidence
Liquid nitrogen	I
Bleomycin	II
Carbon dioxide laser therapy	III
Pulsed dye laser therapy	II
Surgical therapy for condyloma	V
Surgical therapy for plantar warts	V
Electrosurgery for condyloma	III
Electrosurgery and curretage of nongenital warts	III
Interferons	I
Podophyllin for genital warts	I
Cantharidin	II
MCAA, DCAA, TCAA	II
Contact immunotherapy	III
Cidofovir	IV
Intralesional immunotherapy	II
Photodynamic therapy (ALA-PDT)	I
Intralesional vitamin A	IV
Hypnosis	II

Table 19.4 Our recommendations

HPV infection	First line	Second line	Third line
Common warts	Liquid nitrogen in office, salicylic acid at home	Cantharidin	Bleomycin, vascular lesion laser, contact immunotherapy, intralesional immunotherapy
Genital warts	Liquid nitrogen in office, imiquimod at home	Podophyllin 25–50% in office, Podophyllo-toxin at home	Vascular lesion laser, intralesional interferon, intralesional immuno-therapy
Planar warts	Imiquimod	Liquid nitrogen, retinoic acid	Vascular lesion laser, intralesional immunotherapy
Plantar warts	Paring and liquid nitrogen (two cycles) in office, salicylic acid at home	Vascular lesion laser, intralesional immunotherapy	Surgery, bleomycin

published. It is our belief that the information in this book will be obsolete when an effective HPV vaccine is introduced that prevents and treats warts. Unfortunately, we do not foresee a 'cure' in the near future. Some of the barriers to finding an HPV vaccine include the more than 100 types of HPV and the uncanny capability demonstrated by HPV to evade the immune system.

For now, this book provides an up-to-date approach to treating HPV infections. Of course, before initiating treatment, it is imperative to consider whether any treatment is necessary. The best study of the natural history of untreated warts demonstrated that only in 40% of patients did all the warts disappear within 2 years.[9] Therefore, it is more likely that untreated warts will continue to enlarge, spread and become more resistant to treatment. We believe that nearly all warts should be treated with careful consideration of costs, risks and benefits.

Although it is not known whether the risk of malignant tranformation in warts is reduced with treatment, it would be expected that treatment would decrease the spread of HPV because infectivity is related to the number of infective particles in almost all infectious diseases. This may prevent the development of a cancer-promoting infection in contacts.[10,11]

Large warts are cosmetically objectionable and often inhibit function. Smaller warts should be treated as early as possible when treatments are most effective, before they enlarge and spread. Recurrences are common and should also be treated promptly. We are optimistic about the outcome when dealing with our patients. Thoughtful selection of treatments using the vast array presented in this book leads to a clinical cure of warts in most patients. Accepting that most warts should be treated, and that we have imperfect evidence on which to base this treatment, experience and the 'art of medicine' will always play a role in treatment decisions.

The strength of this book is in our attempt to review the literature and critically evaluate the data. We have rated the level of evidence

Table 19.5 Commonly employed therapies for warts

Treatment	Advantages	Disadvantages	Frequency of treatment
Liquid nitrogen	Safe in pregnancy	Scarring, dyspigmentation, pain, variability of treatments	2–4 weeks
Salicylic acid	OTC, cheap	Requires time to achieve response	Daily at home
Photodynamic therapy		Pain (so severe only recommended in adults), scarring, pigment changes	Variable according to study
Bleomycin	Only one treatment needed	Pain during and after treatment, pigment changes, Raynaud's pheno-menon, expected necrotic eschar	Usually one treatment only
Laser (CO$_2$ and PDL)		Scar, pain, cost	Often only one treatment is needed
Contact immunotherapy	Treated at home	Need to sensitize	Daily at home
Intralesional immunotherapy	Only need to treat one wart	Few studies, rare flu-like symptoms	Every 3 weeks
Podophyllin	Painless application	Irritation, teratogen	Every 1–3 weeks
Podophyllotoxin	At home use	Irritation, teratogen	Twice a day for 3 days a week for a maximum of 4 weeks
Interferons	Low recur-rence rate, not destructive	Cost	Two to three times per week
Imiquimod	At home use	Cost, erythema, pruritus, erosions, bacterial infections	Three times a week for EGW

supporting each therapy. These are summa-rized in Tables 19.2 and 19.3. In addition, we have used this information and our experience to make overall recommendations (Table 19.4). Of course, these recommendations are not intended to serve as a cookbook for treatment decisions. There are circumstances in which a third-line treatment might be selected as an initial therapy. We hope instead to assist in decision-making and stimulate thinking about treatment options by bringing data together in one place. Individualized treatment plans for each patient must be tailored to each unique situation.

REFERENCES

1. Lemprière WW. Treatment of warts. *Aust J Dermatol* 1951; **1**: 34–7.

2. Sackett DL. Rules of evidence and clinical recommendations on the use of antithrombotic agents. *Chest* 1986; **89**(suppl 2): 2S-3S.

3. Cook DJ, Guyatt GH, Lamparis A, Sackett DL, Goldberg RJ. Clinical recommendations using levels of evidence for antithrombotic agents. *Chest* 1995; **108**(suppl 4): 227S-30S.

4. Phillips B, Ball C, Sackett D et al. Oxford Centre for Evidence-based Medicine. Printed on website viewed 11 March, 2002: http://cebm.jr2.ox.ac.uk/docs/levels.html. NHS R & D Centre for Evidence-Based Medicine, Oxford.

5. Drake LA, Ceilley RI, Cornelison RL et al. Guidelines of care for warts: human papillomavirus. *J Am Acad Dermatol* 1995; **32**: 98–103.

6. Gibbs S, Stark R, Harvery I et al. Local treatments for cutaneous warts. *The Cochrane Database of Systemic Reviews* 2001; Issue 1 (date of most recent update 16/2/2000)

7. Sterling JC, Handfield-Jones S, Hudson PM. Guidelines for the management of cutaneous warts. *Br J Dermatol* 2001; **144**: 4–11.

8. Wardropper A, Wooley P. Treatment of anogenital warts in genitourinary clinics in England and Wales. *Int J STD AIDS* 1992; **3**: 439–441.

9. Massing AM, Epstein WL. Natural history of warts: A two-year study. *Arch Dermatol* 1963; **87**: 306–10.

10. Quan MB, Moy RL. The role of human papillomavirus in carcinoma. *J Am Acad Dermatol* 1991; **25**: 698–705.

11. Pfister H, Schegget JT. Role of HPV in cutaneous premalignant and malignant tumors. *Clin Dermatol* 1997; **15**: 335–47.

12. Wiley DJ. Genital warts. *Clin Evid* 2001; **6**: 1232–42.

Index

Numbers in italics indicate *tables* or *figures*.